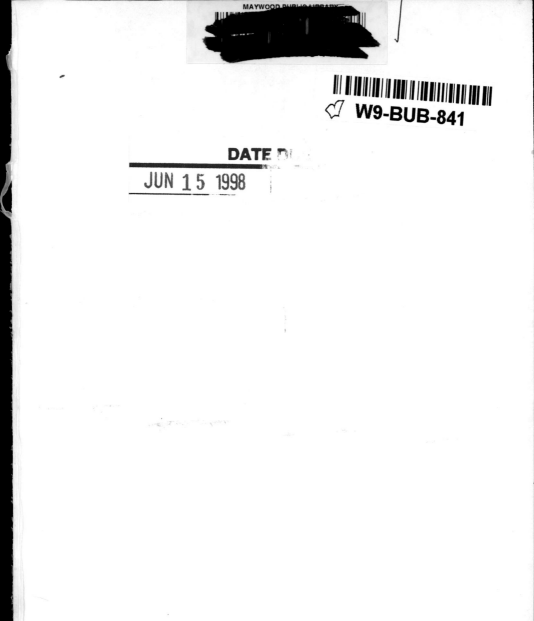

# Looking Down From the Mountain Top

## ....The Story of One Woman's Fight Against All Odds

## by Christine Michael

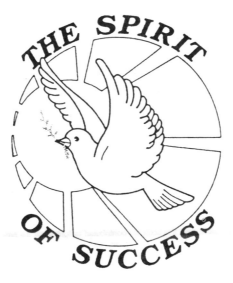

Spirit of Success Publishing Company

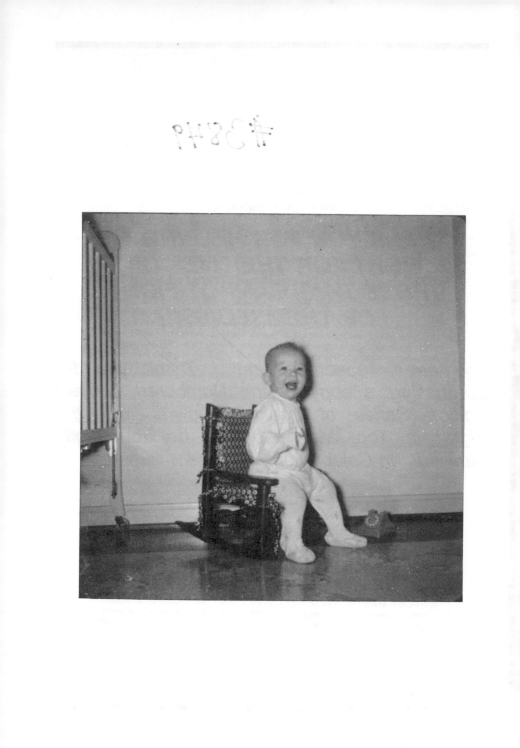

# DEDICATION

This book is dedicated to
**Victor W. Horadam, M.D.,**
the man who gave me the
encouragement to believe
that cancer doesn't have to
mean death, the ability to fight
when there seemed to be no
reason to hold on, and the
support to go on against
all odds.

and

to my precious son.....
**Christopher Michael,**
whom I have never seen, but who
lives with me everyday through
the lives of all of those that I
meet during the Celebration of Life.

and, of course....

to my precious Lord and Savior,
**Jesus Christ,**
for without Him, I would not be
here today.

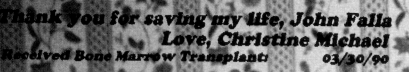

Thank you for saving my life, John Falla
Love, Christine Michael
Received Bone Marrow Transplant:                03/30/90

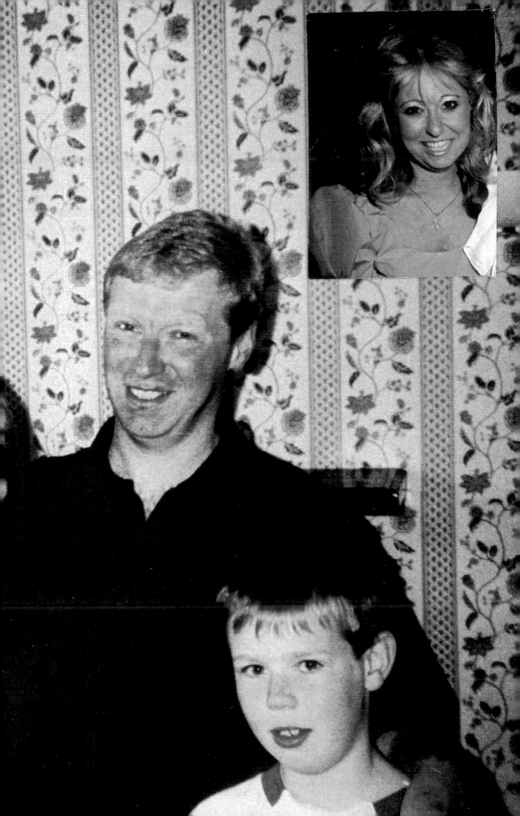

*This is the beginning of a new day*

*God has given me this day to*

*Use as I will*

*I can waste it or use it*

*for good.*

*What I do today is important,*

*because I'm exchanging a day of*

*my life for it. When tomorrow*

*comes, this day will be gone*

*forever, leaving something I*

*have traded it for. I want it to be*

*gain, not loss; good, not evil;*

*success, not failure;*

*in order that I shall not regret the*

*price I paid for it.*

# LOVE LETTER FROM JESUS

*. . . But Jesus said, "Let the children alone and do not hasten them from coming to Me, for the*
*KINGDOM OF HEAVEN*
*belongs to such as these."*
*Matthew 19:14*

*. . . Unless you become as little children - you cannot enter the KINGDOM OF HEAVEN.*
*Matthew 18:3*

*. . . The KINGDOM OF HEAVEN is Within.*
*Luke 17:21*

*. . . Seek First the KINGDOM OF HEAVEN and all these things shall be added unto you.*
*Matthew 6:33*

*. . He that has ears to Hear, let him hear. . .   Mark 4:9*

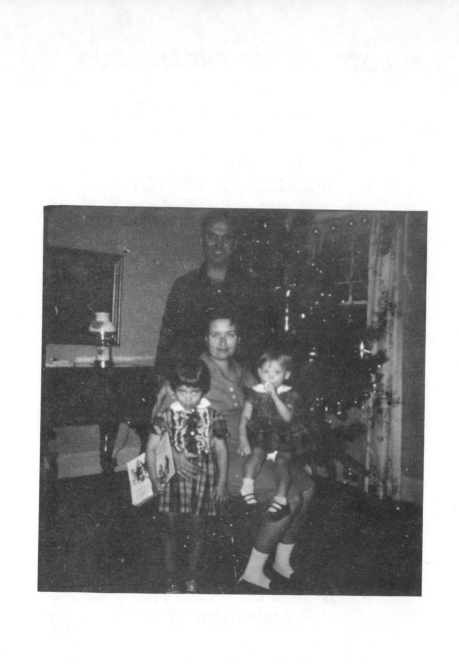

# ACKNOWLEDGEMENTS

To my parents, **Al and Betty,** who taught me that love means many different things. It does not mean always approving of what one does, nor does it mean having to approve of what one does. Human love is not perfect, yet it is always there. Once you have truly loved, you will never stop loving. To my parents, who never left my side. . .you were there when I relapsed with cancer. You were there through the entire transplant procedure and you were there through the recovery process. You gave me support when I did not deserve it. You put up with my endless mood swings and countless bashings toward the people that I loved the most. For that I am truly sorry and I am also truly greatful. You are my shining armor and I love you with all my heart.

To my aunt, **Alma** - who gave me love, support and encouragement during the most painful process of my life. You knew what it was like to lose someone that you loved dearly. Not only did you help me emotionally, but you also helped support me financially when I needed it the most. I love you.

To **Highland Oaks Church of Christ,** whom God used to heal my broken heart. You showed me love in a way that I had never been loved before. You reached out to me by not just telling me about the love of Christ, but you showed me the love of Christ. Your many phone calls, hundreds of cards and letters, and your constant prayers gave me support when I had nothing left. You ministered in ways that helped save my life, as well as the lives of many others. You donated many pints of blood. And you sponsored a bone marrow drive trying to beat the odds of finding a match for my transplant. You hold a special place in my heart.

*"All true prayer somehow confesses our absolute dependence on God. It is therefore*

*a deep and vital contact with Him. . . It is when we pray that we really are."*
*(Thomas Morton: No Man Is An Island)*

To **Vicki,** my very dear friend. You took me under your wing when I had nowhere to turn. You stayed by my side during my crisis and during my battle with cancer. You were there the night that I was diagnosed. You were there during the many visits to my doctor before I relapsed and you held my hand during every bone marrow biopsy. You prayed for me constantly. When I did relapse, you were there with your daily phone calls, your numerous cards and letters and your **bright** colors. I will never forget the night that I became critically ill. For the first time, I did not care whether I lived or whether I died. My mother called you and you immediately came to the hospital. I would not see anyone. You came in without my knowledge. When I saw you, I looked into your eyes and began to cry. I loved you so much and your love for me literally melted my heart. I really believe it was that moment my life began to turn around. You gave me a reason to continue to live. I will always be thankful for that night that I heard the Lord speak to my heart, "Call Vicki and John." I had only met you once, but that was the start of a very special friendship. I love you, Vicki.

To the many churches and prayer ministries that gave meaning to the scripture, "Pray without Ceasing." I know there are many churches and individuals that prayed for me daily that I am not even aware of. To you I am equally greatful. I believe so much in the power of prayer and in the power of the mind. During those times I felt that I was losing the fight, you lifted me up through your faithfulness in prayer. I truly believe that is the reason that I am alive today.

*Psalms 55:16 "As for me, I will call upon God and the Lord Shall Save Me"*

*"I Pray for the progress that is possible when I am completely honest with myself. On that foundation, I can build a good life."*

*"If thou be wise, thou shalt be wise for thyself"*

To **Richardson Heights Baptist Church,** I want to especially thank you for the support you showed my parents during this ordeal. You showed your love through your constant prayers, cards and letters. I thank you so much for the many prayer-grams that I received. I also want to thank **Darrell,** who continued to make trips to the hospital - even though you were never allowed to come in and visit me. You continued to visit daily. You released many pints of blood from your church account for my benefit and distributed materials to increase the awareness for the need for Bone Marrow Donors.

To **Park Cities Baptist Church,** once you have truly loved you will always love. Your continual support and encouragement is greatly appreciated. You constantly sent prayer-grams; for that I am truly greatful. For your phone calls, cards and letters, I thank you. To **Paul** a special thanks. Many times you came to the hospital knowing that you would not be allowed to see me, yet you still came. I can never express how much it meant to me when you came to the hospital waiting room and stayed for hours when I delivered my stillborn son. To **Laurie,** who made sure that I stayed on the prayer list and kept the church updated about my condition You were the one person in my life that was honest enough with me to express your fear, but committed enough to stand by my side and never leave me.

To **Casa View Baptist Church**, for keeping my name in your prayer room and for expressing your love and concern through your continual prayer-grams.

## PSALMS 55:17 *"Evening, and morning, and at noon,*
*I will pray. and cry aloud: and He shall hear my voice."*

To **First Baptist Church of Euless**, for your unfailing commitment in praying for me and keeping my name in your prayer chapel. Your members prayed twenty-four hours a day. I thank you.

To **Metro Prayer Line**, who continued to lift me up in prayer.

To **Highland Park United Methodist Church**, who was so encouraging when I called and asked for prayer from your church. I thank you for the long conversation that we had before I entered the hospital. Often you called to check on my condition. Thank you.

To **Lovers Lane United Methodist Church**, for your endless prayer support and phone calls.

To **Water of Life Church**. You not only stood in prayer for my healing, but also sent ministry tapes to me for encouragement. You served as a constant reminder that I do have a God who truly loves me and wants the best for me.

To **Word of Faith**, who stood believing that the Lord was going to heal me. You continued praying until you saw the manifestations of that answered prayer. To **Ludie** who was God's little messenger, I will never forget you. Your phone call increased my faith ten-fold.

To **Highland Park Presbyterian Church**, for your faithfulness in prayer.

*PHILIPPIANS 1:3 "I thank my God for every remembrance of you."*

To **Central Park Church**, who kept my name flowing through your prayer line and prayed specifically for each need in my life. I saw those specific needs addressed by your church and I saw those same needs answered by the Lord. I thank you.

To **Christ for the Nations**, for the special prayers that you offered in my behalf. For keeping me on your prayer list and for believing that we have a God that is big enough to heal His children no matter what.

To **Calvary Temple**, who had special prayer for me. To the woman that I spoke with on the phone that gave me such encouragement by sharing the testimony of God's healing in your son's life.

*Courage is like love; it must have hope for nourishment*
*Napoleon*

To **First Baptist Church of Garland**, who somehow found out about my story and put me on your prayer list. I thank you for the phone calls and for coming to the hospital to let me know that although we had never met, you knew that God was moving in my life.

To **First Baptist Church of Dallas, Soulwinners, White Rock United Methodist Church** and to the **Baylor Hospital Prayer Line**, I thank you.

To **Saturn Road Church of Christ**, who touched my heart in a very special way. Although we had never met, you had such a burden on your heart for me. You continuously sent cards of encouragement, letters of support and continued to keep me in prayer throughout the year. I thank you, particularly, for your participation in the Bone Marrow Drive at Highland Oaks. You are special. **Lou** . . . , my dear friend. I had never met you, yet you called daily to give me support and encouragement. You reached out to someone that you had never met and provided compassion. I am so thankful that you came into my life.

*"God Dwells Wherever Man Lets Him In"*
*(Martin Buber)*

*For We Walk By Faith. . . Not by Sight*
*(Second Corinthians)*

*"Because a thing seems difficult for you, do not think it is impossible for anyone to accomplish. But whatever is possible for another, believe that you, too, are capable of it." (Marcus Aurelius)*

*"I pray for the wisdom to understand my difficulties clearly and honestly. And for the strength to do something constructive about them. I know I can count on God's help for this." (Al-A-non)*

To **Ross Avenue Baptist Church** and my dear friend, **Roy,** thank you for your prayers.

To **First United Methodist Church of Carrollton**..the choir and church members who continued to pray for me.

To **Fellowship Bible of Park Cities.** . thank you for your commitment to prayer and for reaching out to help find the match for my transplant.

To **Hillcrest Church.** . . you kept me on your prayer list and never gave up believing.

To **Audelia Road Baptist Church,** I know many of you because you prayed for me daily although we had never met. You still call to this day. You have touched my life deeply.

To **Church on the Rock, Cathedral of Praise, Orchard Hills Baptist, Second Baptist of Garland** and the hundreds of others that I could not possibly list... it is because of you - I thank you.

*The possibilities of tomorrow are usually beyond our expectations"*
*Anonymous*

*"To love human beings is still the only thing worth living for; without that love, you really do not live"*
*Soren Kierkegaard*

To my OB/GYN, **Ted E. F.,** whom I have been going to since your first year of practice. You are not only my doctor, but my friend and my guide. It brings tears to my eyes to think about the love and concern that you have always shown me, but particularly on September 2, 1988; the day that we delivered my baby. I will never forget the look in your eyes as you told me my that the baby had died. The next morning when you induced labor you looked as though your heart was as broken as mine. From 4:30 P.M. until 10:30 P.M. that night, you never left my side. You stayed with me during recovery and personally escorted me to the Critical Care Unit. You stayed with me until you knew that I was falling asleep. On Thanksgiving Day, you gave "Joe" and I the keys to your weekend home so that we could have some time alone. You kept me on the prayer list at your church, your family continued to pray for me, and you came to visit me every day. You have touched my life in a very special way and you are one person that I am truly proud to know. To **Peggy,** my true friend. You came to the hospital on your day off and stayed with

"Joe" and I during delivery and recovery. You made it almost a daily practice to come visit me and bring me some gift of encouragement. You diligently prayed for me and had your church choir join in those prayers. I will never forget the first day I was diagnosed with Leukemia. You rushed over to my hospital room even before "Joe" arrived at the hospital. You sat on my bed and your eyes filled with tears. You put your head down and began to cry. You said, "It's just not fair; you have waited so long and he's just a little baby. Why do things like this have to happen?" I began to cry, but I also began to fight. Your honest and sincere love touched me in a way that gave me strength to press on. For that, I will always be thankful. You shared the two most special moments of my life with me. I will never be able to thank you for your love and compassion the night that I released Christopher Michael and began to celebrate my life. I love you.

To **the nursing staff at Presbyterian Hospital** and to **Dr. Horadam's staff. . . ,** I love you all. You are so much of the reason that I got through my battle of cancer. You gave me love, hugs and encouragement during my long term admissions to the hospital. You would come into my room and sit and talk. You would give me encouragement concerning how well I was doing. When I think of you, I think of you as my family. You are all so close to my heart and I love each of you dearly.

To **The Bone Marrow Transplant Staff at Baylor University Medical Center**, I thank you. The ten weeks I spent in the Bone Marrow Transplant Intensive Care Unit was a difficult time of my life. You made it so much easier to endure. Although I do not remember a lot about that experience, I do remember the long talks that we had. All the plans that we made for doing fun things together when I got out of the hospital gave me hope for tomorrow.

To **Kathryn**, who gave me support when my insurance was canceled. You went beyond the call of duty and showed your personal concern for my well-being. Thank you for making a difference in my life.

To **Charter Hospital**, for teaching me how to fight for the child that could not fight for herself. In my case. . . , that child was me.

*"And if by chance that special place
that you've been dreaming of leads
you to a lonely place, find your strength in
love"*
*Michael Masser and Linda Creed*

To **The Housing Authority of the City of Dallas..** there are no words to say - I love you.

AND To **Joseph W. F., M.D.**, who brings a smile to my face when I think of you. You performed my transplant and gave me back my life. I think of the many times that you made me laugh and the many times that you were so optimistic about my recovery. I thank you. You believed in me and caused me to believe in myself.

*"In quiet and in silence the truth is
made known"*

*AND TO WHOM I AM MOST GREATFUL . .*

**John Falla,** *my "anonymous"donor from Scotland,* whom I have never met (at least at the time of this writing),but who I literally owe my life. You sacrificed a part of your life for someone that you had never met. For a person that you had no idea who they were. . .you gave my life back to me The only thing that you knew was that I was dying and that was enough for you. I now have your blood running through my body and your marrow producing my blood cells. You gave a gift that can never be repaid. My prayer is that you receive every desire of your heart. Someday soon we will meet.

## AND A SPECIAL THANKS. . .

To **Arlene Leibs,** who set me back on the path of living life to it's fullest. I love you dearly.

> *"My life is. . . a mystery which I do not attempt to really understand, as though I was led by the hand in a night where I see nothing, but can fully depend on the Love and Protection of Him Who guides me"*

> *Thomas Merton*

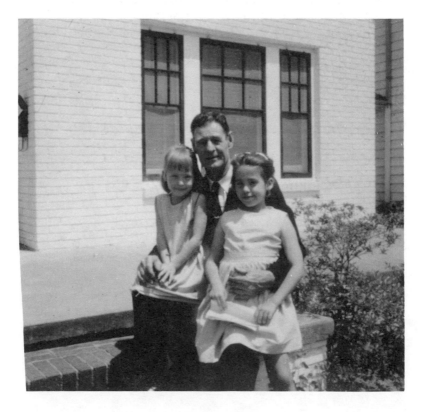

# TABLE OF CONTENTS

_Looking Down From the Mountain Top_ is divided into three parts. Each part is dedicated to a courageous individual who fought the battle of leukemia while searching for a donor to provide the life-saving marrow transplant they needed. The donor was never found. Part I: _Miracles in the Midst of Hell_ is dedicated to David Mayo; Part II: _The Child Within_ is dedicated to David Leibs and Part III: _Celebrate Life_ is dedicated to Ashley Bradford. Each of these individuals will be remembered for their wonderful contributions in this life. They will remain in our hearts forever.

## PART I

## MIRACLES IN THE MIDST OF HELL

# PART II

# THE CHILD WITHIN

# PART III

## CELEBRATE LIFE

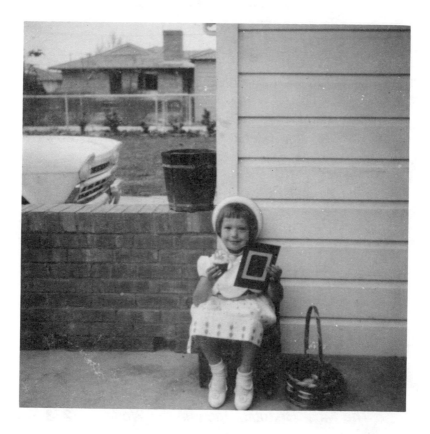

# FROM THE AUTHOR

I have attempted to write this book for the past two years. It seemed as though every time I neared completion, the ending kept changing.

I never understood why. Now, I know. I have learned so much in the last few years. I have learned about myself, about the true meaning of love and mostly, I am learning for the first time in my life how very much our God truly loves us and wants the very best for each of our lives.

My prayer is that every person that goes through the struggle of cancer or the heartbreak of an ended marriage or the devastation of losing a child will search within themselves to find the answers. As human beings, we have a tendency to search outside for the reasons for life events. But what I have found through my experience is that the answers lie within ourselves. It is within our own heart. The peace comes from within and this is my prayer for each of you who reads this book.

I have lost everything that a person could lose in this lifetime, but I have gained so much. I am happier than ever. For the first time, I have found that the love I was so desperately searching for was the love within; the love for myself.

In the words of Denise Lachance, a graduate of Arizona State University, who was once a resident of Girlstown, U.S.A. . . . she wrote and I echo:

# TO EACH OF YOU

who through very change I encountered
patiently awaited my fumbling recovery.
waited until my childish tempers lashed out at those
who loved me too much to defend themselves
You listened to my endless tales of woe and tribulation
although I never stopped talking
cared and counseled
when I never stopped hating and hurting.
You were willing to see things in me
I could not find in myself and had not the unselfishness
to seek in others
You presented me with pleasures you had tasted
hoping that one of us, at least, would find some of the
answers and helped me bear the pain I
was too weak and empty to carry for myself even
though your own trials were weighing you down
seemingly to the very core of the earth.
You, who did not disrespect me
when I lacked any respect and all compassion
I had no trust in your friendship then, even as
I ached with every shred of being to love and be loved.
Each of you, my true friends
must find me greatly changed
older perhaps, wiser I hope. do not be disturbed for
in the peace that I have finally
found for myself, I have discovered
empathy and trust.  This is a peace that I need to share
with Each of You, because I Love You.
I do not bear a yoke of troubles around my neck, but
neither will I expect you do to this for me any longer.
One who lifts all burdens does this for me.
Yes, you may think me greatly changed, but I hope
so much easier to love.

# *PREFACE*

"Mommy, Mommy. . . ,please don't give me away!!" How those thoughts terrorized my mind as a child. I never quite understood what I had done that was so wrong. It seemed as though no matter what I attempted, it just wasn't quite good enough.

I remember many times my sister and I would be playing. We would get into fights, as young siblings often do. I would hear my mother pick up the phone and say, "Is this Buckner's Orphan's Home? I have a little girl that doesn't know how to behave. We don't want her anymore. Can you come get her?" My sister and I would scream in fear only to be comforted with, "Alright, then, you better behave!"

My dad was my idol. I truly thought the man knew everything. I could ask him any question. He would know the answer to it. I wanted so much to please him and have him love me. I never felt as though I was good enough. I would be so excited about a major accomplishment in my life. I would rush to share my latest discovery with my dad. My reward would be his monotone reply of, "Well, that's good." My little heart would be crushed. I wanted him to share in my excitement. Most of what I heard, if I ever got up the courage to question his lack of enthusiasm, was "Sweet-heart, you have so much potential. You're just not using it. You could do so much better." Of course, my heart would sink. Once again, I had failed.

I learned very quickly that to receive love I had to be the **best**. So, I set out to prove to everyone around me that I was the best. I learned to behave in a manner and to play the role of a "perfect" three year old. I never understood exactly what that meant, but I knew as long as I was "performing" I would not be given away. When I didn't quite hit the mark, and I had one of those tantrums that pre-schoolers are so skilled at having, I would hear my mother say, "Now, Christine, would Jesus love you if you did that?" I would reply with a broken heart, "No, Mommy."

I loved Jesus with all my heart. Why couldn't He love me? It wasn't long before I learned to hide all my faults. I would pretend that I was an incredibly happy child. I soon found that my smile could open most doors. When I entered elementary school, I learned that my smile would win friends and would make people love me the way that I wanted to be loved. Of course, they could never see any of my faults. Then the game would be over. I would be right back where I started from. . . . . . .unloved and unwanted.

I was so confused. I knew that if I let go of my facade, then people would see me for who I really was. Then. . .they wouldn't really love me and I would be left all alone.

The struggle went on for many years until, one day. . . I found my "miracle." It was a miracle in the midst of Hell, but it was one that truly changed my life.

# *Miracles in the Midst of Hell is dedicated to*

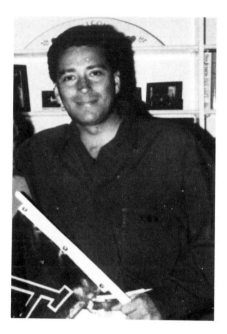

# **David Mayo**

**who lost his battle to Leukemia
while searching for a donor
Born:  August 16, 1958
Died:   October 8, 1990**

# PART I

# MIRACLES IN THE MIDST OF HELL

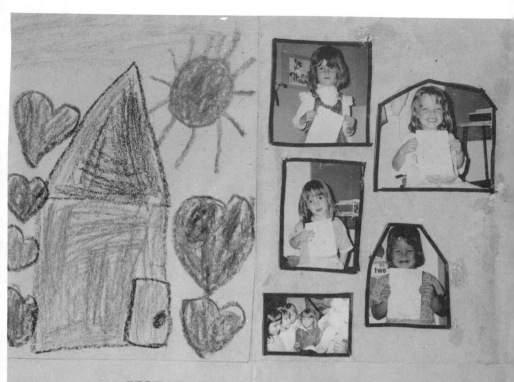

**"PLEASE FIGHT FOR US. . .
WE CANNOT FIGHT FOR OURSELVES"**

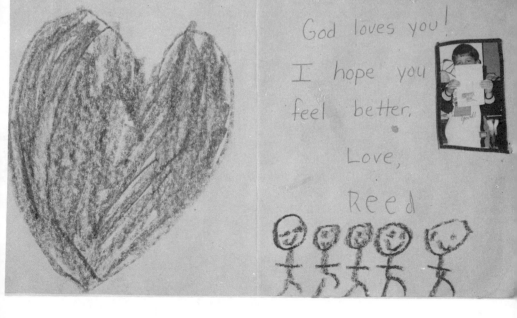

God loves you!
I hope you
feel better.
Love,
Reed

# CHAPTER ONE

## Until Death Do Us Part

If you have ever been to a place where all your dreams came true, where every particle of your being radiated with the fulfillment of your innermost desires and with each breath you took, you felt as if you were going to be lifted off the face of the Earth, then you have been to the mountain top. That is where I lived in 1988.

I was in love and I was getting married to the man that I had looked for my entire life.

Before I met Joe, I had lost faith that my dreams would ever come true: finding that "perfect" life-time partner and having the baby I so desperately wanted. After struggling with an eight-year relationship that came to a painful end, I had given up hope.

But everything changed when I started dating Joe. I met him where I worked - a low income housing development agency with the City of Dallas. At first I was mesmerized by his looks: his handsome face was punctuated with blue eyes that seemed to smile on their own, his salt-and-pepper gray hair, his athletic build and his natural charm made him totally irresistible.

But as I got to know him, I discovered something that was even better than the "packaging." He seemed to understand my pain and disillusionment caused by the events in my life. As we grew to know each other in a very intimate way, we discovered that the bond we shared had a lifetime purpose: raising a family in a loving and nurturing environment which neither Joe nor I had experienced growing up.

We fell deeply in love with each other. We thought at the time that all the hurt from the past would somehow disappear if we were together. We were strong Christians and we truly believed that with God's help, we could conquer anything.

The wedding I had planned came right out of my childhood fantasies. I would wear a white satin wedding gown and the longest cathedral train I could find. All the bridesmaids would be dressed in red velvet and the groomsmen would wear black tuxedos with red bow-ties and red cummerbunds. The Christmas candlelight ceremony would have a very spiritual tone as we dedicated our lives to each other and to the Lord who brought us together. My sister would be my maid of honor, since she had always "stood by my side." She understood what it was like to be thirty and not married. My dad would give me away before the groom and I knelt to take our vows "until death do us part." My parents would be so proud of me.

As the wedding day approached, my dream was starting to take shape. The church was reserved. The hotel ballroom was awaiting the magical evening of dancing and celebration. Red roses and baby's breath were ordered to fill the church.

About five weeks before the wedding, my sister called me and said something that broke my heart: she was dropping out of the ceremony. I immediately called my mother in tears and told her the bad news.

I thought someone had stabbed me in the heart with a knife when I heard my mother's reply. "Well, I don't blame her," she screamed. "I think it's ridiculous to have that big of a wedding. I'll tell you another thing, too. If she's not there, your dad and I aren't going to be there either. Furthermore, we're not paying for it."

My dreams had been destroyed.

I called Joe in hysterics and asked him to come over. I laid in his arms and cried. He reminded me that the wedding was not the most important thing...it was that our vows were taking before God.

Trying desperately to comfort me, he said, "No matter who is there, even if it is just us, it is still a sacrament. It doesn't change the relationship."

Three days later, Joe and I "eloped" through the yellow pages. We got married at a minister's house with four close friends as witnesses. During the ceremony, I fought back the tears as I thought about my "dream wedding" that would never happen. I never went to pick up my wedding gown from the bridal shop. It was just too painful.

Although I was devastated from the failed wedding plans, I filled my time trying to create a cozy homelife for Joe and myself. I decorated our Mesquite home with primitive antiques, woven rugs and a sentimental collection of country folk art. We spent many nights on the deck or in the hot-tub talking and making plans for the future.

We had not been married long when I discovered that I was expecting my first baby. Twenty-two weeks of pregnancy went by so quickly. It was hard to believe that in a few short months I would have the precious baby that I had waited for so long to have. I still remember that overwhelming emotion of lying down at night to suddenly feel that little life inside of me - a life that Joe and I had created and a life that I had dreamed of for so many years. I often tried to picture what my baby looked like at each stage of development. I would try and imagine what he was doing when I felt him move. Was he stretching out? Was he curling up and sucking his thumb to go to sleep?

I was so happy the first time Joe and I heard the baby's heartbeat. Somehow that little life represented the new life that Joe and I had found in each other. I loved lying down to go to sleep and feeling that precious life depending on me for its life.

I never knew that it was possible to love something so deeply that I had never seen. That life inside of me had somehow become the most important thing in my life. Now I had both things that made my life complete. I was married to the man that I had waited all my life for and I was expecting our first baby. I was truly living on the mountain top.

It was a hot morning in August--one of those mornings when everyone complains about the heat and humidity. But I woke up feeling incredibly happy to be alive.

As Joe continued to sleep, I went into the bathroom to get dressed. It was at that moment my heart almost stopped beating.

I screamed to Joe: "Joe, my God, I'm losing my baby. I'm bleeding." Joe jumped out of bed, called the doctor, and rushed me to the hospital. The thirty-minute drive to the hospital was not long enough to change the intensity of my crying. I just kept praying, "Lord, please don't let anything happen to my baby."

As we got off the elevator in Labor and Delivery, and as I put on the hospital gown, I felt my lips start to quiver with fear. The nurse came in to hook me up to the fetal monitor. She asked me: "Is this your first baby?" I nodded as tears rolled down my cheeks.

She quickly made her own diagnosis. "Well, there is nothing wrong with this baby...this baby is perfectly fine! He's got a strong heartbeat and he's moving around all over the place."

I was so relieved. From then on, I didn't hear a word that was said to me. I entered my own little world of communion with my son.

I was startled out of my hypnotic trance as the doctor reached out and touched my arm. He asked me a few questions, but I could hardly hear him...I was watching the incredible miracle of life inside of me being charted on the monitor.

The hospital ran some more tests, and they discovered the origin of my bleeding: I had an extremely bad kidney infection. I was sent home and told to rest, A huge wave of relief washed over me.

The next day I got up and was taking a shower with Joe, as we often did together. I was shaving my legs when he said, "Honey..." and reached out to touch my leg. It was pouring with blood. I had barely nicked myself.

As I was getting ready for work, I lightly scratched my face. It began to bleed and it wouldn't stop. I constantly blotted the wound, but two hours later in my office, it was still bleeding. I knew something was terribly wrong.

I called Joe immediately, but he wasn't home. I called my dad and asked him to meet me at the hospital. As we were waiting for the results of the blood tests, it seemed like every doctor and nurse that walked by was looking at me strangely - as if they knew exactly what was wrong.

The minute I saw the doctor's face, I knew we were going to get bad news. He said he was going to admit me to the hospital for some more tests; that the results of my blood test were not normal. He would refer me to a specialist to make sure, but it appeared that I had leukemia.

When he said the word "leukemia", my entire body went numb. I was too afraid to ask questions.

Thank God my father was there. He asked the question I didn't want answered.

"Doctor, what about the baby?"

"I'm sorry, I'm afraid we'll have to terminate the pregnancy." After the doctor said that, it was as if I were watching myself in a movie on television. I heard the words, but I couldn't relate it to myself.

After we left his office, it suddenly seemed that the entire world was filled with expectant mothers. I turned a corner and almost ran over a precious toddler. I looked down at him and said, "Hi, Sweet-heart," as my eyes filled with tears. I grabbed my stomach trying desperately to feel that life inside of me.

That night we checked into the hospital room. I didn't know it at the time, but that room would become my home for many months. My dad called Joe to tell him the bad news. As Dad handed me the phone, I started to cry. Hearing Joe's voice on the phone gave me strength. He said he would get to the hospital as soon as he could.

He was there in just minutes, and the oncologist, Dr. Douglas, wasn't far behind. The doctor said I would need a bone marrow biopsy to confirm the leukemia. As he explained the procedure, I kept waiting to wake up from this horrible nightmare.

As I lay in the hospital bed having the biopsy taken, I started to laugh. Two phrases kept going through my mind. One of them was a Bible verse: "I can do all things through Christ who strengthens me," and the other was "What do you say about a 25-year old girl who died?" which is the opening line of <u>Love Story</u>--a book and a movie where the lead character dies of leukemia. I think it was the absurdity of those two phrases that kept me laughing.

I told my doctor: "I believe in the power of prayer, the power of the mind and the power of modern medicine. When you put these three things together, you have a true healing power. Now, it was time to find out if I really believed the words that flowed so easily off my lips.

The biopsy turned out to be definitive: I had a rare type of leukemia called acute promyelocytic leuke-mia. The leukemia was so advanced, 98% of my blood cells were malignant. But that wasn't all I had: I had another disease called DIC (disseminated intervascular coagulation) that prevented my blood from clotting.

Dr. Douglas explained that the difficulty in having both of these diseases together was that the treatment for DIC worked against the treatment for leukemia. Add to the fact that I was pregnant, and I presented a real catch-22 for my doctors. If they treated the leukemia - it could harm the baby and result in my death. But if they didn't, I would definitely die.

As if I hadn't heard enough, I asked the dreaded question again: "What about the baby?"

There was no way they could terminate the pregnancy, Dr. Douglas explained, because I would bleed to death.

In some strange way, that gave me hope. There was no way I could have chosen to terminate my pregnancy - I would have literally died before I could give them permission to take the life that I had grown to love so much.

Because my doctor had never seen a case like mine, he said he would contact experts at leading cancer centers across the country, and by consensus, they would decide the best treatment for me.

He said that under normal circumstances, I would have an 80% chance of getting my leukemia into remission. But in my case, he wasn't sure if they could get me into remission. "If not," he said, "You are looking at about six weeks to live."

After I heard that, the elaborate structure of prayer, medicine and positive thinking collapsed into a heap of total denial. I kept thinking, "I must be dreaming...this can't be happening." Joe and I spent the evening together in each other's arms. I didn't cry until Joe left the hospital. I didn't want to waste a minute of our time together."

I had said to friends on many occasions, "If Joe ever died, I would be dead six months later." I knew that I loved him enough to die for him. I just hoped I loved him enough to live for him.

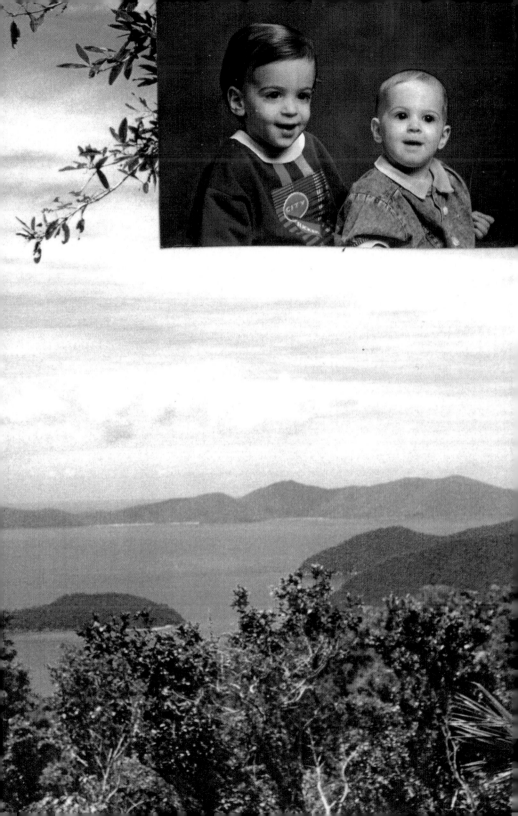

I love you,
God loves you too.

Love,
BlaiR

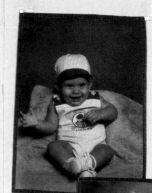

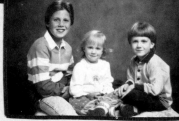

**PLEASE FIGHT FOR US. . .**
**WE CANNOT FIGHT FOR OURSELVES"**

I LOVE YOU

# CHAPTER TWO

## The Call To Fight

After Joe left, I lay totally alone in the dark and I tried desperately to find a way out of this nightmare. There had never been anything in my life I couldn't control completely - now I was completely powerless.

At that point, I began to cry out to God from the bottom of my heart. "God, please, I am begging you..I don't want to die. For the first time in my life I am truly happy. I want to live."

I was lying in the fetal position trying to protect my baby, although I knew I was powerless over his life, too. It was then that I felt a presence in the room. I stopped crying and stared into the darkness. I saw a vision of Jesus hanging on the cross. His head was hanging down and then he looked up at me. A tear ran down his face. I heard a voice within me say, "I will never leave you, nor forsake you. I love you."

It was as if Jesus was telling me that He knew the pain within my heart and He knew what it was like to face death. Although He was God incarnate, He was also a man who loved me so much that he gave up His life for me.

I quickly reached over and turned on the light. I grabbed my Bible and turned to the Old Testament and read about a king who had been given a prophecy that he was going to die. The Bible verse said, "The Lord heard his cry and said, 'because of your faithfulness, I will add 15 years to your life.'" I felt as though the Lord was speaking to my heart.

Another thought came into my mind. It was that of my supervisor at work, a loving man who had such a positive influence in my life. When I had told him earlier that day that I had leukemia, he said, "Well, Christine, you are always so positive. Now it's time you practice what you preach. Remember... whatever the mind can conceive, the body can achieve." I recited this like a mantra until I finally fell asleep.

The next morning was my call to fight. Armed with my strong Christian beliefs and my "mind-over-body" mentality, I was ready to take on just about anything.

My oncologist was the first person I saw that morning. He was very direct and honest when he said: "Christine, we have decided to treat your leukemia very aggressively. There is a great risk that your baby may die in the process - and with the DIC - you would bleed to death. But we have no other alternatives."

Every word he said after that seemed to raise my level of anger by one degree. He talked about the transfusions I would need and the possible side effects. He talked about hair loss, weight loss and mouth ulcers.

As he talked, I wanted to say: "Don't I have enough to worry about? How do you know exactly what is going to happen to me? You just met me!"

Instead of asking him questions about the side effects, I just barreled right on through to my little "presentation." I told him that I believed in visualization - a process where you picture in your mind what you want to accomplish. I told him I believed in the power of prayer, mind and medicine.

He said he thought my philosophy was great. . as long as I didn't use it by itself. But it was missing one thing. "Medicine can only do so much and after that...you just have to have a sense of humor."

Although I didn't know it at the time, we had found a common ground that would see me through my battle. We both shared the incredible love of laughter. The relationship that we formed truly set a healing force in motion.

From that point on, I started to see the positive side of my disease. I actually looked forward to my chemotherapy and treatment for DIC. I could apply the many principles of motivational training which I used in my seminars to my illness.

Since I was not allowed to leave my room, and since I couldn't have any guests, I had time to devote my full attention to relaxation exercises. I applied "guided imagery" techniques to my body - I pictured all my blood cells coming together and forming clots. I pictured my cancer cells being eaten up by a massive dose of chemotherapy.

But that week, my imagery and relaxation techniques were no match for my body. Not only was I nauseated from the chemotherapy, I started to gain weight and get excruciating headaches. With the added weight of the baby, I had ballooned up to three times my normal size and I could barely breath.

My doctors suspected that I might be hemorrhaging from the brain, or that I had a brain tumor. Even though I was in unbearable pain, they didn't want to give me excessive medication to control the pain because it could harm the baby. But if they didn't give me any medication, the situation would get worse and cause my death.

The more symptoms that appeared, the more determined I became to win this battle. I would start to name the things that I had to be thankful for. I called this process, "One step, alleluia, Jesus!"

I would say, "I'm thankful that the brain tumor tests were negative...I don't have a brain tumor....alleluia, Jesus!"

Although I couldn't stand any light in my room, I reached for the phone book and began to call churches that had prayer ministries. I didn't care what denomination they were. If they believed in prayer, I wanted to be on their list.

I continued my visualization techniques. . .with each new complication, I tried to visualize the desired result.

My motivation through this entire ordeal was my baby. I constantly stroked my stomach and tried to comfort him. I would tell him, "Hang on. Mommy loves you."

But suddenly one day, for some reason, I stopped talking to my baby.

My headaches got worse and I developed debilitating back pain. My doctor ordered a sonogram to check for internal bleeding. As the lab technician administered the test, I noticed no movement on the screen. I immediately chalked up my fears to ignorance. I asked the technician, "What about the baby?" She replied curtly: "Well, they really didn't ask me to look for that."

Back in my room, I glanced outside the hospital window, and saw my obstetrician, Dr. Duckett, walking across the parking lot toward the hospital. Before I had time to dismiss my fear, he was opening the door to my room. He had tears in his eyes. "I don't know how to tell you this..." he said. My baby had died.

Joe had not planned to come to the hospital until later that night, but for "some reason" he decided to come early. He was in my room only seconds after the doctor had told me the bad news. I didn't cry that night. I just kept trying to feel my baby move, but there was nothing.

My doctor told us that I could continue to carry the baby for another month before my body would go into labor. It was a strange comfort to keep the baby inside of me. My doctor sent Joe and my parents home and said, "There is no reason for you to stay. She may not deliver for weeks. However, if her body decides to abort tonight, she won't make it through the night."

I took a sleeping pill, but it did no good. All I could do was stare at the ceiling and see pictures of my baby that I had so vividly created in my mind.

It was 3:00 AM when the lab technician came to draw my blood as she did every night. My doctor came in the room a few hours later and said he was "shocked" by the results of the test. The DIC had "miraculously" disappeared. He decided to waste no time and induce labor that morning.

The next day at 6:30 PM, after 12 painful hours of labor, I delivered a stillborn baby boy. During labor, my blood pressure skyrocketed and I developed partial paralysis - both of which the doctors fought hard to overcome. When the baby's head began to crown, the anesthesiologist knocked me out so I never saw my baby. To this day, all I have are the pictures I created in my mind.

I was taken to the Critical Care Unit after recovery. I was awakened by a nurse who said, "I understand that you just got out of delivery. Where is your baby? Is he in the nursery?" I answered her with tears rolling down my face. I replied, "He's dead'".

Joe was with me through the entire ordeal. When I woke up in the middle of the night, I realized he had gone. Feeling something wet, I reached down to touch my hospital gown. As nature takes care of its own, milk was seeping from my breasts to feed the life it had created. I buried my face in my pillow and cried myself to sleep.

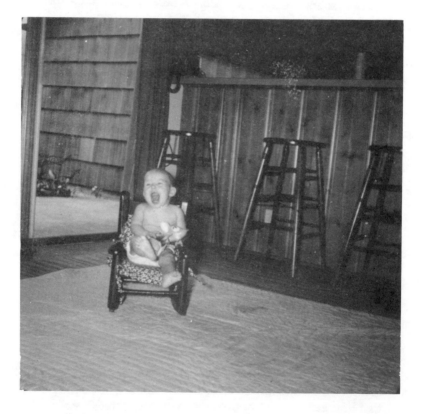

# CHAPTER THREE

## The Angel In the Candy Store

I didn't have time to grieve as it was back to the battlefield the next morning.

Within a day of delivery, all of my weight began to disappear and my blood pressure returned to normal. In retrospect, my doctor realized that it was "eclampsia" that was the cause of my weight gain - the only cure for this fatal disease is delivery of the baby.

I was overwhelmed by my "miracles in the midst of hell." I had three life-threatening diseases and God had delivered me from two of them. After going through that ordeal, the rest of the struggle seemed easy. I became an "ordinary" leukemia patient with 98% cancer cells in my blood.

That morning, the oncologist did a biopsy to determine the status of my leukemia.

When he came into the room that afternoon, he had an almost bemused expression on his face. He said he couldn't see any leukemia cells, although the pathologist felt sure that there must still be some.

"If that's true," he said, "that's the first time I have ever seen that during my practice. I responded with a smile, "That's the first time you've had Christine Michael and her God as a patient!"

Even in my most fearful time, I continued to pray and claim victory by visualizing all my cancer cells turning into healthy cells. And my doctors continued to be amazed at the results of my bone marrow tests. I told everyone I was stuck in the middle of a miracle. We all tripled up on our prayers and I tripled up on my visualization techniques.

Looking out the window of my hospital room, I watched the leaves turn color and realized that Thanksgiving was not too far away. I wanted to badly to spend the holiday with Joe and just celebrate our lives together. I felt I had been to hell and back, but I had so much to be thankful for. As I started to think about the gifts I had been given, another prayer was about to be answered.

The phone rang and the voice on the other end said, "Christine, you don't know me, but I am well aware of who you are. I really don't want you to know who I am since I work in the hospital." This woman continued to explain, "When I first saw your name come up on the computer, God placed such a burden on my heart to pray for your life. I didn't know what was wrong with you. All I knew is that I was supposed to pray for you. My church had a special prayer service for you.

"Since then, I have found out a lot more about what you are going through. I have felt so called to intercede in prayer for your complete healing. I have wanted to see you, but the sign on your door. . .'No Visitors'. I did not know what to do. This morning, I got up and felt so impressed to call you and tell you to be encouraged; God loves you, Christine...He's healing you. You are going to be fine! The Lord has a special purpose for your life and He is going to use you in a mighty way," she said.

As this woman was reaching out to me, I was alarmed by a loud noise. It was Dr. Douglas flying into the room with a beaming smile on his face. He said, "Do you want to go home now, or do you want to go home in five minutes?" I don't believe it, but your leukemia is in complete remission. There are absolutely no signs of cancer cells!"

Although he released me from the hospital, I had to return for two more rounds of chemotherapy. He said I should be out of the hospital by Christmas, but I told him I wanted to be out by Thanksgiving. So he made a deal with me. He said that if I didn't have fever or infections, I could go home by Thanksgiving. But he saw that as an impossibility.

I saw it as a challenge. I wanted more than anything to spend Thanksgiving alone with Joe - we hadn't even had time to grieve the loss of our baby. It had been months since we had been able to hold each other and kiss - much less make love.

I watched my temperature drop during that week and by Thanksgiving Day, my counts were normal.

Before I left the hospital, I fantasized about the perfect place to spend Thanksgiving. There was a Christian encampment close to Tyler, Texas, where I used to stay when I traveled for business. Set back in the piney woods on a lake, it is one of the most beautiful places I have ever been. You can sit for hours and not hear a sound except for the birds and the gentle wind brushing through the tall timbers.

I phoned the secretary of the encampment and explained my situation to her. She said Thanksgiving Day was free, but there was a conference the next day. It worked out perfectly.

I was so excited that I called my parents immediately with the good news. I felt like the same little girl who always tried to share my excitement - just once I wanted to hear them say, "Honey, that's wonderful!" Instead, I heard my mother say, "You're doing what??? I can't believe you're doing this to your family. After all we've been through, you're not even going to spend Thanksgiving with your family."

I began to cry. I said, "Mom, I have not been with my husband in over three months. We have not even had time to grieve over the death of our baby. Please don't do this to me."

As usual, there was no understanding from my parents. And as usual, Joe said, "Honey, why do you continue to set yourself up?" I couldn't understand what he meant. I just wanted to spend Thanksgiving with the person that made me happy. It seemed so simple.

That day was a turning point in my life. I did not understand why my parents always seemed to be "bursting my bubble." But I did start to see that no matter how hard I tried to get their approval, it would never happen.

I started to analyze my entire life through this experience. No matter how much I hurt, I would always smile. It was as if I was standing outside a candy store and I wanted desperately to buy a loaf of bread. I stood there year after year, with my nose pressed against the glass, hoping that someone would sell me a loaf of bread. I had all the candy I wanted, but none of it seemed to matter because that was not the real desire of my heart.

Like the "good little girl" I had always been, I broke down and spent Thanksgiving Day with my family. All during the day, I watched and I listened. I listened to the family from whom I had sought love for so long. Every time one of them said something that hurt me on the inside, I saw the candy store. I knew I never could receive love and approval from the people I wanted it from the most. I could stand there until eternity passed, but the bottom line is they just don't sell bread at a candy store.

When I was still in the hospital, my good friend Dr. Duckett came to visit me. I told him about the encounter with my mother.

He asked me, "What if you had a place to go the day after Thanksgiving?" He offered me his private lake home, surrounded by an acre of woods that was nearby the conference center. I gladly accepted.

As we drove up to his home, we looked on the other side of the deserted road. There was a long hidden driveway that led up to the conference center. The rustic atmosphere was perfect for a romantic get-away.

We unpacked the car, and I felt Joe become a little distant. When I asked him what was wrong, he said, "Nothing," but I knew differently.

We decided to go to the store and buy some food for breakfast. As we started to leave for the store, Joe turned around and asked me, "Where are you going?" He looked at me as though he were trying to hide something.

"Stay here. I'll go to the store and when I get back, we can have breakfast."

At that point, I felt like a small child who was being told to stay in the car while their parent went grocery shopping.

"That's okay," I responded, "I'll go with you," as I started to walk towards the door.

I heard Joe's voice screaming back at me: "Damn it, just stay here!" I could not believe what I was hearing; he had never acted that way before. But the more I protested, the angrier he became. Naturally, being a "good girl", I stayed in the house.

When Joe returned, he was all love and kisses. But I couldn't hide my tears.

"Are we going to start this again?" Joe said with a definite edge in his voice.

I said, "Joe, I feel like I just walked into the 'Twilight Zone'. All I wanted was to go to the store with you." After twenty minutes of confrontation that made absolutely no sense to me, I said. "I don't understand. I love you and I thought we were here to spend time together."

We sat down at the breakfast table. It was so beautiful with the sun shining through the tall pine trees. I thought, "Why can't things just be the way they are supposed to be...I'm so tired of being hurt."

As I looked into Joe's eye's, he grabbed my hands and began to talk. He said, "The first night you were diagnosed with leukemia I cried for hours. It was such a strange feeling. . .I had only cried once in the past 20 years. I went home and I told God, 'I am so afraid to lose her. I am begging you, please don't let her die.. she is everything I have ever wanted.'"

He continued to talk.  My heart broke as I listened. "You lose the baby, and I can't do a thing for you. I don't have a job, so I can't support you. I start thinking it would have been better if I had never come into your life - you would be a lot better off without me."

Long after the Thanksgiving get-away, this conversation lingered in my heart. I started to remember that he had said very similar things on a visit to the hospital after the baby died. And I remember when we were dating, how painful it was for him to open up to me and show the pain of his past. I wanted so badly to try to help him, to reach inside his broken heart and say, "Baby, it's okay, I'm not going to hurt you." But what I didn't know at the time was all the desire on my part could not change who Joe was on the inside.

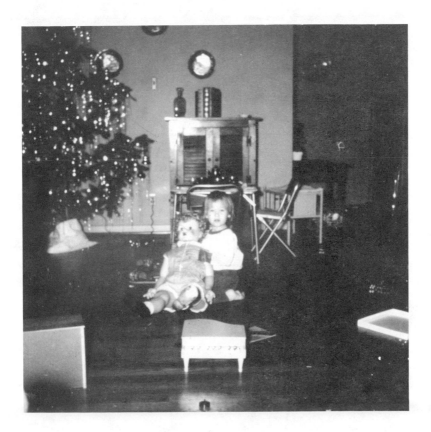

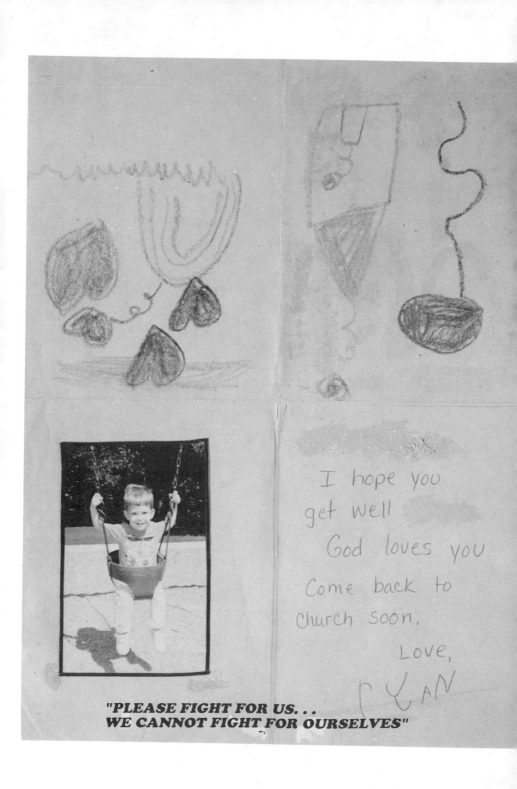

I hope you get well
God loves you.
Come back to church soon,
Love,
RYAN

**"PLEASE FIGHT FOR US. . .
WE CANNOT FIGHT FOR OURSELVES"**

# CHAPTER FOUR

## The Candy Store Robbery

The mission to save Joe became my main focus in life. Every time he withdrew, I pushed him to open up. He tried to open up and we became more and more intimate. I saw so many positive changes in Joe. We started getting involved in the couples class at church instead of just going to the worship service as we had been doing. He seemed to be finding a piece of himself that had been missing, and at the same time he was losing the fear that plagued him. We had been apart for so long - it was as if we were on a second honeymoon. We would take long walks and sit and talk for hours.

Joe and I had a very active and passionate sex life before I got ill. It was as though no two people were more sexually compatible than the two of us. The passion and the feelings had always been overwhelming to both of us. Somehow, this day was more special than I could have imagined. It was also more difficult than I could have imagined.

As we were sitting on the couch in the living room, Joe reached out and took my hand. He looked into my eyes and he didn't have to say another word. We walked into the bedroom. As he began to kiss me, I felt my whole body turn inside out. It had been so long since we had been together, but he still took my breath away. He pulled me next to him and began to kiss my neck. As I lifted my head toward the ceiling and closed my eyes, all I could think about was how very much in love with him I was. As he gently laid me across the bed, I looked into his eyes and stroked his face with my hand. As we started to make love, I began to cry.

It is so difficult for a woman to feel desirable - no matter how much a man tells her he loves her or how many times he tells her that she is beautiful - when she does not believe it herself. Somehow when you have scars on your body from IV needles, scars on your breasts from a catheter and you are pale from chemotherapy - you just don't feel very desirable.

All I could think about was: "What if my wig comes off? Who wants to make love to a bald woman?"

Somehow Joe and I got through that first time. He got angry because I cried, and I cried because ha got angry. But we were still together. Over time, our sex life got back to normal.

And the rest of our life gradually got back to normal too. It was mid-December when I was told I could return to work in just a few weeks. Joe would be starting a job on January 3 - the same day I would return to work. Ironically, it was the same day that our baby was due to be born had he not died. God was opening the door for a new life together, far more beautiful from having gone through this experience.

The brief normalcy was interrupted after I had been back at work only two days - I returned to the hospital for emergency gall bladder surgery. I was out of work for six more weeks.

When I finally did return to work in mid-February, I started doing volunteer work with the Leukemia Society of America. Along with other concerned citizens, I started a group called "Life-Link," a non-profit organization that would raise funds for tissue typing and increase awareness of the need for bone marrow donors. I started working with cancer patients to teach them how to cope with their disease. The more involved I became, the more I learned what a miracle it really was for me to be alive.

It was at that time I started to see a purpose in my life: I did not want others to have to go through the pain that I had gone through.

I noticed that my deepening involvement with cancer patients and surrounding issues was really starting to bother Joe. I remember one day Joe and I went out to eat. We ran into a couple from our church. I had never met this man's wife. The man introduced me as "the woman I was telling you about." He told his wife what a miracle it was that I was alive and that I had been diagnosed with leukemia. I talked about the changes God had made in my life and my new "mission" to help cancer patients. We got out to the car and Joe lambasted me about my comment. "Why can't you just give it a rest?" he asked. "It's over!! Why can't you just go on?"

This time I became irate. I said, "What am I supposed to do? Am I just supposed to say, 'Well, thanks God' and go on? There are **thousands** of people dying from this disease each year. We are less than five years away from a cure. . . a **CURE**, Joe! Am I just supposed to sit back and not give a damn about any of those other people? I can't do that! A large number of those lives that we are losing are children, Joe! There is no reason why anyone should have to die of leukemia anymore!"

Joe and I would often have the same argument. Joe wanted to bury it and I just could not do it. I feel that when things happen in someone's life, they don't necessarily happen for the best, but they can be used for the best if we choose to let them.

Our relationship was great as long as we did not discuss the past or talk about anything that was painful. So I buried myself in volunteer work and my job, and Joe was busy with his new job. It was the last week in March before our next crisis hit.

Joe was out of town on business. He had called me and said that he was heading out to West Texas to make some cold calls. He told me that he would call me when he arrived and let me know where he was staying. The phone rang and I ran to answer it. I missed him so much when he was out of town.

To my surprise, the voice on the other end was not Joe's voice. It was Joe's son, Richard. He told me that Joe's mother had died. I explained to him that his father was on his way to West Texas, but I would try to find him. After calling every hotel in West Texas, the phone finally rang. It was Joe's voice on the other end of the line. He was crying. He had found out about the death of his mother. He kept saying, "Baby, I can't believe she's dead." It was suicide.

Joe blamed himself for the death of his mother. I encouraged Joe to call her when he was in her town the week before. Joe had just started speaking to his mother again before we got married. I used to tell him, "Joe, life is too short. You don't have to be the best of friends, but at least open up the lines of communication."

He had called her. She begged him to come see her. He told her, "Mom, I'll come see you next week when I'm in town." He did not tell her that he was just a few miles away from her house. Three days later, she committed suicide.

Joe continued to cry on the phone. He kept repeating, "I can't believe that my mom is dead!" He told me that he was on his way to pick up his daughter in Dallas and that they were going to drive to his mother's house in Houston. I told him, "Baby, please don't drive to Houston like this. It's late and you're upset. I'll drive you down there, Sweet-heart." At that point, he instantaneously stopped crying and there was a deafening silence on the line. His voice tone changed abruptly. He became cold and distant. He said, "You're not going. I'm going to go pick up **MY** daughter and go to **MY** mother's funeral and **YOU'RE** not going."

I knew when Joe told me how his mother died - my life was going to be "hell." That night Joe completely shut me out. He just kept pushing me away emotionally. Joe had taken all the pain he could stand. I think that I could have found Joe in bed with another woman and it would not have hurt me as much.

Late in the evening two days later, I heard the front door open. I usually ran down the stairs when he came in from out of town and threw my arms around him. This time I was frozen. I couldn't move. I could not believe that I was so afraid of my own husband. He had opened the scars of my past and for the first time, I was truly afraid of being hurt by him. The man that I knew was the one person who would always love me, I was no longer sure would always stay with me.

Joe came upstairs and I pretended to be asleep. I didn't know what to say to him. He had something in his hands. He went into the bathroom and put it down. Then he came back and stood by the bed - just staring at me. I could barely hold back the tears as he made his next move. He took my wrist in his hand and felt for my pulse. I was "sleeping so soundly" he thought I had left him too. . .just like his mother. He leaned over and gave me a kiss on the forehead and left the room.

When I finally mustered the courage to follow him, I found him on the day bed in the guest room. He was sitting in the dark - staring into space.

He said, "So, I'm going to kill you, too." He never looked up when he said it and he did not say it as a question or with any defense. He said it as though he really believed it. I said, "Joe, what are you talking about?"

He said, "I killed my mother."

When he made that statement, I didn't care if he did kill me. I could not stand to see the man that I loved immensely and who wanted so much to be loved - be in such pain. I sat down on the bed. I put his face in my hands and said, "Sweet-heart, you didn't kill your mother. She committed suicide. Honey, once someone has decided they want to end their life, there is nothing that anyone can do. They are going to do it!" We talked for hours. He seemed to reach out just a little; just enough to let me hold him.

He said, "We need to go down there this week-end and take care of the estate and clean out some stuff."

I said, "You mean you and your daughter are going down there?"

He looked at me and said, "No, I mean you and I need to go down there." He proceeded to say, "Honey, I don't know what is wrong with me. I just didn't want you to be a part of that crap. When I met you, everything in my life changed. Somehow I just felt that if you were exposed to that, you would become a part of it. That was wrong though. You are my wife and I love you. You need to be there. I need for you to be there."

We went upstairs and I saw what he had left in the bathroom. He had bought me a new Evan Picone suit and a dozen long stem red roses. He had also brought me a rose from his mother's casket. I said, "Don't you want to keep this rose?" He told me that he wanted me to have it because I was a part of his past. His past was a part of him and he was part of me. If he only knew how much.

If it is possible to love someone too much, I was guilty as charged. With Joe coming from a dysfunctional family of alcoholics, I knew that deep down all that he needed was to be loved. I had waited all my life for someone to love me just as I was; not for what I was or who I was. I felt that I had found that in Joe. I knew that Joe and I had made progress. Joe was not going to push me away, or so I thought.

Joe never really got to know his real father. Since he was an alcoholic and could no longer handle Joe, Joe's father had shipped him off to his grandparents and had very little contact with Joe. His mother had deserted the family when he was a young child. During Joe's junior high years his mother reentered his life and wanted to renew their relationship. He moved in with her and her husband. Joe grew to love his step father immensely. I think if it had not been for the influence that this man had on Joe, Joe probably would not be alive today.

Joe and I went to the reading of the will that weekend and went to his mother's house in Houston to start cleaning up. We would have to put the house on the market. Because of the constant moving around as children, Joe never got to know his sister very well. Now there was a chance for a reunion, because his sister lived in Houston. Joe told his sister that we would be coming in town every weekend. We would help paint and get the house ready to sell. We never made another trip down there. Every weekend that we had plans to go visit, Joe would come up with some excuse. He always said, "We'll go next weekend." Next weekend never came.

Three days after we came home from his mother's house, in a matter of an hour, Joe was fine. It was as if his mother never died. It was scary how Joe could literally turn off his pain. It was like it never happened. Joe handled his mother's death as most people would handle the death of a pet. Most people would cry for a few days and get over it. That is how Joe handled the death of his mother. He did no more grieving and refused to talk about it by saying, "It's over."

I knew that Joe was dying on the inside. For the first time in our relationship, I couldn't reach him. Before the death of his mother, even when he pushed away, I could eventually get to him. This time was different. He had gone to a place that I didn't know how to reach. It was as if he had a deep dark hole at the depth of his being. He had let someone in for the first time, but now he was shutting the door.

The next couple of months grew more intense. Joe was traveling three days a week. Everytime he came in from a business trip, I could tell that he had been drinking. Joe never drank during our relationship and we never kept alcohol in the house. For the most part, when we went out, Joe would order iced tea.

Although I was in the field of human resources and worked with an employee assistance program, I was so wrapped up in my own denial I could not see that Joe had his own disease. . .a disease called alcoholism. I tried to encourage him. But the more I reached out, the more that Joe pushed away.

Having my own insecurities from childhood and having a constant fear of being abandoned by anyone that really knew me, I was finding it difficult to hold on and to continue to take risks with Joe. I felt as though I was constantly walking on eggshells. Every time that Joe lashed out or when he pushed me away emotionally, I would "put on my smiley face" that I had learned to do so well as a child. I knew that if I was "good enough" Joe wouldn't leave me.

The dark hole deep within Joe became the foundation of our marriage. We both tried desperately to hold on to each other. It became a vicious cycle: the

more we held on, the more we destroyed each other.
Welcome to the disease of addiction.

Amidst the pain of my relationship with Joe, my
health seemed to be improving.  Although there were
stressors in my life, all my reports were coming back
positive.  There was no sign of leukemia, yet my odds of
survival were only 50%. That was good enough for me.

My oncologist was constantly talking with me
about the need to look for an unrelated marrow donor
since I did not have a match in my family.  He said "I
want you to go ahead and start a search for a donor.  If
your leukemia ever does come back, then we'll be
ready.  If it comes back and you don't have a donor
search begun, there will be nothing we can do. It takes
a while to find a donor and I'm not willing to take that
risk for you."

I made an appointment with the doctor who
does the bone marrow transplants in Dallas: Dr. Mike
Mitchell. He was a big, friendly teddy-bear of a man, but
he was a very serious doctor. He explained why I would
need a transplant if I relapsed: my bone marrow was the
source of all my blood cells and immune system cells.
Because my blood cells were defective - through the
leukemia - my bone marrow had to be replaced, or
transplanted. He said that having an unrelated donor
was showing the best results; however, an unrelated
donor was extremely difficult to find. The chance of
finding a matched unrelated donor is 1:20,000.

In the meantime, he wanted to harvest some of
my own marrow while it is healthy; just in case I couldn't
find a donor.  "We treat your marrow with the same
chemicals as we treat you," he explained. "So, just in
case there are any leukemia cells in it - if you ever
relapse, we give your own marrow back to you." "It's a
fairly simple procedure," he continued to explain.

I was so tired of hospitals and being stuck with needles and being put to sleep. I wanted so desperately to be "normal" again and to have my marriage "normal" again. For some reason, I got extremely afraid of going to the hospital. Dallas Community Hospital - where I had all my previous surgeries and treatments - had become my home. I knew all the nurses there and we had become good friends; I knew no one at Metro University Medical Center. Although it has an excellent reputation, I did not want to be there. The "harvest" was scheduled for May 1, 1989 at 7:00 A.M. I asked Joe to take me to the hospital. He acted as though I was asking him to give up his only son. He told me that he had an important meeting in Louisiana that he could not miss. I said, "Joe, can't you call and ask them to postpone the meeting?" He wouldn't hear of it.

He said, "It took me forever to get this job and now, you want me to just 'blow it off'?" I didn't want him to "blow it off." I just wanted him to be there while I was having my marrow harvested.

I told him, "Sweet-heart, you don't have to stay. I realize the harvest is not that big of a deal. It only takes about thirty minutes. This is not actual surgery and I'll be out of the hospital by 2:00 P.M. this afternoon. But for some reason I am scared to death. Can't you wait until they put me to sleep and take me to surgery and then you can leave?" He agreed to try and postpone his meeting. He called the buyer and asked if they could meet at a later time. There was a later flight that Joe could take if he changed airlines.

That's all I wanted. Joe and I got up the next morning to go to the hospital. He seemed extremely nervous. I asked him if he was okay and he said everything was fine. But, as it had been the last month, I felt as though I was sitting with someone that I didn't even know. The wall between us was so thick that it literally felt like I was suffocating from lack of air.

I hope you feel better. Hope your hospital rooms O.K.

Love,
Chase

"PLEASE FIGHT FOR US...
WE CANNOT FIGHT FOR OURSELVES"

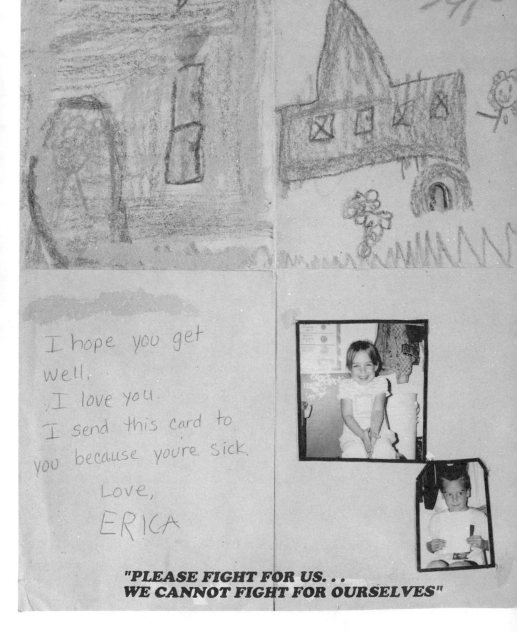

I hope you get
well.
I love you.
I send this card to
you because you're sick.

Love,
ERICA

**"PLEASE FIGHT FOR US...**
**WE CANNOT FIGHT FOR OURSELVES"**

We arrived at the hospital at 5:30 A.M. to check in. The harvest would not be for an hour and a half. Joe had told me that his plane left at 8:00 A.M. He would have to leave around 7:00 A.M. to check in and get his ticket. As hospitals usually function, 7:00 A.M. came and I had not even been taken to pre-op.

Of course, Joe had to leave. My dad had not arrived at the hospital yet, but Joe was insisted that he had to leave. Right before he left the hospital, he asked the nurse, "Doesn't she need to take off her rings and jewelry before she goes to surgery? Joe had given me a beautiful 2.25 carat solitaire diamond for an engage-ment ring. It was my "dream ring." It was simple, yet elegant and so represented our marriage in my mind. I always hated taking that ring off. I had put it on for life and that's where I wanted it to stay. . . for life.

The nurse said, "I'm glad that you noticed that." Christine, you need to give him that ring so he can take it home. We have a place up here, but I wouldn't trust it."

I questioned Joe about his trip to Louisiana. He said, "Well, honey, I'll be home tonight." It will be safe until then. I'll wrap it up and put it in my brief case. It stays locked." I agreed and thought nothing of it.

I got out of the hospital at approximately 3:00 P.M. that afternoon. They had taken a hyperdermic needle and withdrew marrow from my hipbone. I felt like I had fallen on the ice, it was no more painful than that. Dad and I went out to eat as soon as I was released from the hospital and I was back at work the next day. It was so easy, I wondered why I had been so afraid. Joe returned from his business trip the next day and everything was wonderful.

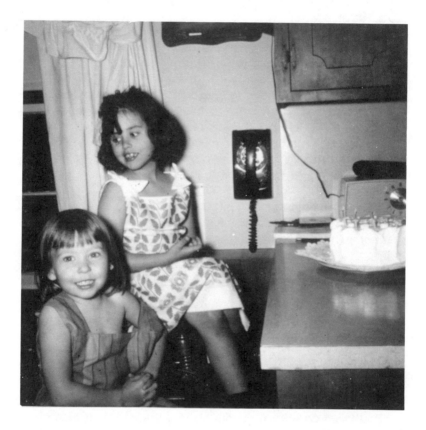

# CHAPTER FIVE

## The Missing Puzzle Piece

After being single for such a long time, I had some definite preconceived notions of marriage. I believe that when two adults are both working and have successful jobs, they should split household expenses, yet maintain separate accounts.

That is what Joe and I did from the time that we were married. Since we did have separate accounts, I never looked at his checkbook.

But by accident, that changed when I rehired my housekeeper to clean my home. I will never forget one Saturday morning that she was tidying up my office. She handed me a bank deposit statement for $8000.00. I knew that I had not made a deposit for that amount and I knew that Joe didn't have money to make a deposit of that size. I looked at the date of the C.D. deposit. My body became numb from shock. The deposit slip was dated May 1, 1989. That was the day that I was in the hospital having my bone marrow harvested.

Joe had gone to the health club to work out while the housekeeper was cleaning. He came home after she left. When he opened the door, I had the C.D. deposit slip in my hand. He came over and gave me a kiss on the back of the neck. I asked him how his workout was although I never turned around to look him in the eyes. He said, "It was great" and continued to tell me how good he felt.

While he was talking, I turned around, looked him straight in the eyes and said, "Joe, where did you get this? This is a deposit for $8000.00. His face looked as though he had seen a ghost. He just stared at me and didn't answer. I repeated my question and Joe looked down at the floor.

He finally said, "I got it from my mother's estate. She left me the C.D." I had been at the reading of the will and didn't remember any C.D.'s being left to us. I did remember that we had a discussion with his sister concerning his mother's financial condition. She had gone through all of her money within the last six months. All the C.D.'s had disappeared. She had apparently cashed them all and spent the money.

That was not even my concern. "Joe," I said, "I'm not talking about the money. We both have separate accounts. I don't care about the money!! What I'm talking about is the date. You made a deposit on May 1st. That is the day that I was in the hospital having my bone marrow harvested. Remember . . the day that you HAD to catch a plane at 8:00 A.M."

"You could not get your meeting changed and couldn't even wait until I went to surgery. The banks don't open until 9:00 A.M., Joe. And this deposit was made in Mesquite! You didn't catch a plane. You lied to me. You didn't even have a meeting."

He looked at me and reached out to put his arms around me. I pulled away. I finally let loose my anger on Joe.

"Joe, you promised me before we got married that you would never lie to me. I love you, but I will not put up with you lying to me. I can handle anything if you are honest with me. You stole money out of my account while I was in the hospital. On more than one occasion, I wrote checks and gave them to you to pay my bills. You didn't even mail them. You took my Pulse card and withdrew the same amount of money for which the checks were written. We're talking about my house-payment, Joe!   They could have foreclosed on our house."

Joe got defensive.  "Well, that's not my idea of a marriage," he said.  "My idea of a marriage is a team. When one partner is down, the other one is there to pick them up.  It's not taking count of who's doing what," he said.  Joe always knew what to say to make me vulnerable to him.

Joe knew that he had gotten to me.  He pulled out all the stops.   He began to get tears in his eyes. "Honey," he said as he put his arms around me, "I just can't stand it anymore.  I am tired of seeing you sick. And I am so tired of being afraid.  I just could not go to the hospital that day.  I feel like if I have to take you to the hospital one more time, I won't make it.  I can not stand it anymore!"

It seemed as though five days out of the week, our marriage was completely blissful.  We had wonderful times together; we talked and laughed.  The other two days were "hell on earth."  So many times, Joe would blow up for no reason.  It would be the smallest of things that got him upset.  He would knock over a glass of tea and would suddenly behave as if he had absolutely no control of his behavior.  Many times he would comment, "What's wrong with me?  I can't do anything right!  !  !  I'm such a failure!"

The angrier Joe became. . .the more I reached out to him.  My attempt became futile as Joe withdrew more deeply into himself.  I would often tell him what a wonderful man he was and how much I loved him.  His reply would be "Yeah, well you shouldn't!"

Soon, I began to see more drastic changes.  Joe and I spent much of our spare time together since he traveled three days a week.  We had a standard evening ritual at our house.  Joe would call me at work and want to go out to eat that evening. He would tell me what time he would be home. I would run home from work only to sit and wait for forty-five minutes to an hour with no sign of Joe. When he finally did arrive, I would run out to the car to meet him and throw my arms around him. He would smile and give me a big hug. Then, he would lean down and give me a kiss that had the stench of a brewery.

I couldn't believe it the first time that it happened. Joe occasionally had a couple of beers when we went out to eat, but it was an exception to the rule. Now, it seemed as though he couldn't make it home from the airport without stopping at a bar during the afternoon. He rarely came home intoxicated, or at least he rarely acted as though he was.

Joe and I had many long conversations about his drinking. I knew that both of his parents had been alcoholics and Joe was a "sitting duck" for the disease of addiction. I told him, "Sweet-heart, you are so vulnerable to alcoholism. There are some real danger signs in your life. It seems like everytime I ask you, you have been to a bar by yourself. It's one thing if you are going out with brokers and buyers for a drink, but sitting in a bar by yourself concerns me."

It was always, "Yeah, I know, but I only had two drinks." I totally believed him when he told me that. Why shouldn't I? I trusted the man with my life and he NEVER came home drunk. If he was late, he was never more than an hour late and most of the time, he was home quicker than that. As women often tend to behave during a crisis in which they are at risk, my concern turned into harassment. Every time he was late, I knew that he was in a bar. We would have a confrontation leaving both of us miserable.

I decided to try another approach. I told him, "Baby, I don't care what time you come home; you can stay out until 2:00 A.M. if you want, but at least call and let me know that you are okay."

That sounded reasonable to him. Joe began to call whenever he was running late. He would leave me a message that would sound something like, "Honey, I'm at the bar with a couple of buyers. I'm about to leave. I'll be home in about half an hour and then we can go get something to eat. I love you." Either there is a time zone difference from one side of our town to the other, my clocks were wrong, or else Joe's promises were becoming mere words. The more resonant his promises became, the more he never followed through on them.

Each day, my insecurities from my own childhood were being brought to the surface of my mind. What had I done wrong? Why didn't Joe love me the way he used to? For the duration of our relationship, Joe sounded like a doting parent telling me how much he loved me. Now, it was the highlight of my day if he would just show up when he said he would. My fear of abandonment was increasing daily. Joe knew me inside and out. I was afraid that I had been right all along. If someone really knew me, they wouldn't love me. They would leave me.

The following month was filled with loving moments trying to hold on to each other. Yet, at the same time we were pushing every button that the other one had trying desperately to make sense out of the madness that we had created in our marriage.

I had talked for months about having a baby. I so desperately wanted a child. I thought, "If I could just have a baby, I would be fulfilled and then Joe could do whatever he wanted." I think I had gotten to the point that I really believed that. There were several times during that month that I personally packed all Joe's belongings before he came home. I had full intentions of telling him to find someplace else to live. The hurt and pain that Joe was inflicting in my life was becoming unbearable.

Joe and I had some terrible fights during the month of July. Everytime I brought up the subject of having a baby, Joe would make his normal comment, "You just want a baby, you don't care anything about me. I know you. If you have a baby, you'll leave me just like everyone else has." Although the thought had crossed my mind, I knew that I could never leave him. Despite how painful the marriage had become, my feelings were so deep and I was more in love with Joe than I had ever been.

We decided that I would try to get pregnant in December. That would be one year from my last treatment. Since I had been doing so well, I felt confident that everything would be fine. The closer that the time came to having a baby, the more excuses Joe made He wanted to put if off until February. . . then April. . .
It was in July that I was late in starting my period. I was the type of woman that could look at her watch and know exactly when she was going to start. I was never late. However, that particular month I was three days late in starting. Joe and I were not getting along well, but our active sex life never ceased. That seemed to be the only time that we could really communicate.

Joe and I had gone out to eat that evening. I told him that I had not started my period. His comment could not have hurt more if he had stuck a knife in my stomach. At first he laughed. He looked at me with intense hatred in his eyes, gritted his teeth and said in a demonically intense tone, "THEN GET RID OF IT!!!"

I felt my heart stop beating. I looked at him and said, "There is no way in Hell that I would EVER get rid of this baby!" I started to cry. "How in the name of God can you say that after you spent twelve hours in labor and delivery with me and our baby **died**, Joe?"

I knew there was something extreme going on with Joe. He had the puzzle piece that I didn't have. Whatever was going on with him had nothing to do with our love for each other. It had nothing to do with our marriage. It had to do with Joe himself. I still searched for answers, but mostly blamed myself for not being good enough. Deep inside, however, I knew there was more to the story. It seemed as though a minimum of three times a week I was on the floor in complete hysterics crying from the fights that Joe and I were having or crying over his constant promises and constant disappointments. He had become so cold, yet at times he would cry and tell me how much he loved me and how afraid he was of losing me.

I will never forget one of those times. It is the day that I call "the day that I nailed the coffin shut on my marriage." Joe and I had a great week. He seemed to really be trying to make an effort to communicate. It was a Saturday morning toward the first of August. Joe was going to take his daughter to lunch. He gave me a kiss and told me how much he loved me. He said, "If Richard calls, tell him that I'll be home around 1:00 P.M. and to come on over." Richard, Joe's son, was in town for the weekend.

It was such a beautiful day. I spent most of the morning in the yard, relaxing in the jacuzzi and waiting for Joe to come home. It seemed as though no matter how bad things were, I still couldn't wait to see him. I remember thinking about that fact while he was gone. I knew that our marriage would always last, because no matter what. . . when it came down to the bottom line, we were very much in love. The more I thought about Joe, the more I couldn't wait to see him. One o'clock came and naturally, he wasn't home and naturally, I received no phone call. I decided that I was not going to get upset.

Every hour that passed, I continued to choose not to be upset. The concept worked in theory, but my blood was boiling on the inside. I looked at the clock and it was 4:00 P.M. By 5:00 P.M., I was ready for war. I knew that Joe had been drinking. All I could think about was, "What if he had an accident?" It always amazes me how I could be so concerned about him that I was ready to kill him.

Finally, around 8:00 P.M., he came rolling in the house with a smile on his face like everything was just the same as it was before he left. He walked over to me and gave me a big kiss. He said, "Hi, Honey. Have you eaten?"

I decided I was not going to get upset. It seemed that all I did was make Joe feel worse about his behavior. It wasn't enough that he already felt guilty. I had to make sure that he felt even worse. This time, I was not going to do that.

"How was your day, Sweet-heart? Did you and Heather have fun?" I asked.

"Yeah, I took her and a friend of hers out to eat and then they wanted to go to Six Flags, so I took them over there," he replied.

I tried not to be defensive and concentrated on asking my questions in a very calm tone. "Sweet-heart, do they not have phones at Six Flags?", I asked. He knew that I was upset. "Joe, couldn't you have at least called me and just let me know that you were okay? I was really concerned about you. You told me to tell Richard that you would be home at 1:00 P.M. and it's 8:00 P.M.!" When a person is desperate, they will resort to all kinds of things. I resorted to down-right lying. "Richard has been here all afternoon waiting for you. Honey, he was so disappointed. He was just in town for the day. He finally left to go back to Austin."

Joe felt badly and was disappointed that he had missed his son and I felt better since the heat was not on me. This time, it was Richard who was upset about Joe being late. Although in reality, I had not talked to Richard in several weeks.

As ritual dictated, Joe came over to give me a kiss. He must have known that he was in trouble because the kiss was deep and passionate. . .and reeked with liquor and Binaca breath freshener. I pulled away and looked at him. "Joe, when did they start selling alcohol at Six Flags?" I asked.

He laughed and said, "They don't sell alcohol at Six Flags!"

"Then, why do you smell like a brewery that has been flooded with breath freshener?" I inquired. I was becoming angrier with each response he gave me.

"I don't smell like a brewery. I haven't even had anything to drink. Let's go get something to eat," he said. He headed toward the door.

"Okay," I said, "but tell me about your day first. Did you'll have fun?" We proceeded to talk about what they had to eat and about how crowded the lines were. As he continued to give me detailed information about his "Disneyland-Daddy" day at Six Flags, the moment of truth came.

I asked him, "What did you'll ride?" I thought that was a simple question. Since he had just spent the entire day at Six Flags, surely he could remember what rides he had been on. He hesitated for a long time before answering.

"Well, we didn't ride anything," he told me.

I said, "You took two thirteen-year-old girls to Six-Flags and you'll didn't ride anything?"

"Well, they rode a bunch of stuff, but I just kind of walked around. They took off by themselves and I had them meet me back at a certain time. You know how that goes," he said.

With great amazement and a concern for his boring day of "just walking around", I said, "You didn't ride anything, Honey?" I knew that I was on a roll.

"Well, I rode the Shock-wave by myself and I drove the cars," he replied. He thought he had me believing every word.

"Oh, the Esso cars?", I asked. He nodded in agreement.

"The ones that they took out in 1963, Joe?" His face went completely blank. I couldn't help but laugh. And of course, he **jumped** on the opportunity to laugh also. The laughter did not last long.

"Where did you go, Joe?" I asked in an interrogatory manner. I gave him a chance to answer, but he did not reply. I somehow remained calm, but I was not going to allow this battle to go on one more day. It was either going to be settled that night or it was not going to be settled at all. I had reached my limit. I knew that I could not continue living as we had been living. It was destroying me. I repeated my question. I looked Joe straight in the eye and said, ".Joe, you <u>promised</u> me that you would never lie to me and you promised me that you would <u>never</u> go to a bar by yourself again. . .Joe, where were you?"

From then on, it was like a game of cat and mouse. He told a story, and I caught him in every lie. Finally, when he told me he bought a few beers at the convenience store, I asked him to produce the empties. When he couldn't do that, I asked him to drive with me to the convenience store to identify the clerk at the store who sold him the beer. He made up a description of a "fantasy" store clerk - and I finally caught him in his big lie when the store clerk turned out to be male instead of female. He finally admitted that everything he had told me that day had been a big lie - that he had not been to Six Flags with his daughter and her friend, but had spent the entire day in a bar.

At that point I knew the truth about Joe - a truth I had been trying to deny for months. Joe was an alcoholic. I was deeply in love with Joe, but I was beginning to realize that no matter how much you love someone - it just doesn't matter if they don't love themself.

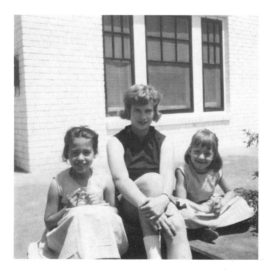

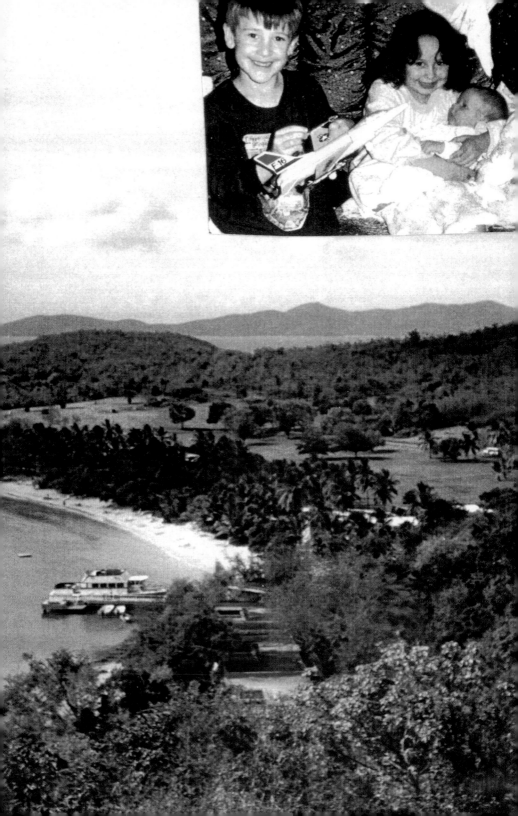

# CHAPTER SIX

## The Final Straw

As we pulled up in front of the house after the "convenience store episode," Joe put his arm around me. I twirled around to get out of his embrace. I escalated my pace to be two steps ahead of his so that he could not touch me.

He started to walk upstairs toward the bedroom. I called after him, "Where are you going?" He stopped in route, but didn't turn around.

"I'm going to bed," he said.

"No, Joe! I will **not** go on another day like this. I can't," I told him.

He came back downstairs. He said, "Baby, I love you. Let's go to bed. We can talk about this tomorrow." Joe kept reaching out trying to put his arms around me. I was like an abused child. Every time that he got within three feet of me, I would escape to the other side of the room.

After approximately one hour of saying absolutely nothing of importance and making no progress toward a solution, Joe started to leave. He said, "We'll talk about this tomorrow. If you don't want me here, I'll go stay in a hotel. We'll talk about this in the morning."

From the look on my face and from the tone of my voice, Joe knew I was serious. I said, "Joe, you walk out that door and you have made your decision. There is no such thing as tomorrow. Joe, tomorrow never comes! By the time tomorrow gets here, it's today."

He somewhat smirked at my comment and said, "Yes, there's always tomorrow."

For the first time all night I was not avoiding being close to Joe. I walked right up to him, got directly in his face, pointed my finger at him and repeated, **"You walk out that door and you have <u>made</u> your decision!"** I then added, "Joe, you stay and you stay on three conditions and three conditions alone: Number one, you quit going to bars by yourself and you quit lying to me about where you've been; Number two, you call me if you are going to be late, and Number three. . . we go to counseling."

Joe was frozen with his hand on the doorknob until I said the third condition.

"No way," he said as he started to walk back into the den. "I'll do one and two, but I will **not** do three. I'm not going to go and have somebody tell me how bad I am."

My heart broke; not only because he said that he would not go, but because I knew that he was in such intense pain.

"Nobody's going to tell you how bad you are, Sweet-heart. They're going to help us," I said.

I could never handle feeling Joe's pain without having my own stance threatened. Inevitably, I would start to crumble. I wanted so much to hold my position.

"No way," he said.

I asked him, "You are willing to give up our marriage and willing to lose me because you won't go to counseling?"

"If that's what it takes to keep you," he said, "then, yes." He was pacing back and forth, but stopped when he made that comment. He looked at me from the corner of his eye - as to make sure I had not taken him seriously.

It was almost midnight and we had been going in circles for four hours. I was tired and I felt like I had been run over by a truck. Out of frustration and out of exhaustion from maintaining a position that was very difficult for me to uphold anyway, I finally said, "Joe, I'm not asking you to stay in counseling. I'm not even asking you to open up to the counselor. I'm just asking you to **go**, to just give it a chance."

He looked toward the floor and then looked at me. "Alright," he said, "I'll go, but don't make the appointment for this week. Make it for next week."

"That's all I want," I said. I could feel the love for him beaming through my eyes. He grabbed me and held me close to him.

"I love you so much," he said.

I began to cry. This time Joe didn't yell. He didn't get angry. He took me by the hand, we walked upstairs and we made love as if we both knew that it would be one of the very last times that we would share the deep love that bound us together.

I woke up feeling a little scared and extremely vulnerable. But I was so thankful that Joe had agreed to go to counseling. He was not going out of town that day, so I was up and dressed before he woke up. When I came back into the bedroom, Joe was awake. I sat on the edge of the bed and leaned over to kiss him. I asked him, "Are we okay, Joe? Are we friends?"

"What do you mean, 'Are we friends?'" he asked. "I love you; you're my wife. Of course, we're okay." He then said he wanted to take me somewhere special that night. He was going to work in Dallas and he'd be home around 5:00 P.M.

I said with a smile, "And what are you going to do if you can't be here by 5:00 P.M.?"

"I'll call you," he said, "but I'll be here."

I was like a little child waiting to go to the circus. I thought about Joe all day. I called home and left several messages saying, "I know you're not there, but I just wanted to tell you 'I love you.'" I couldn't wait to get home. The traffic was somewhat heavy that afternoon, so I didn't get home until 5:30 P.M. Joe wasn't there. I ran into the study to listen to the message that he would have left me. All I heard was the sound of my own voice saying repeatedly, "I know you're not there, but I just wanted to tell you how much I love you."

My body went numb. "Surely not," I thought to myself. Joe said that he wanted to go someplace nice, so I took off my suit and put on something a little more dressy. I freshened up my makeup and went to watch the news on television. Three hours later, I was still sitting by myself staring at the wall.

At 9:00 P.M., I heard the keys in the door. I knew that Joe had been drinking because it took him at least three minutes to get his key into the keyhole.

"Hon-e-e-y. . .," he called out. I don't know how anyone can manage to slur one word, but he managed. He walked into the downstairs bedroom where I had the television on. If someone had asked me what I watching, I could not have even told them, although I had been sitting there since 6:00 P.M. "You're all dressed up," he said. "You look pretty." He walked over to where I was sitting and leaned over to kiss me. He reeked with alcohol and he could barely stand up. I pushed his face away as hard as I could. I got up and went into the den.

As Joe followed, I saw that he had tears in his eyes. For the first time in our relationship, I didn't feel sorry for him. I didn't want to hold him. I wanted to "beat the hell" out of him. I wanted to make him hurt the way that I had hurt. I lost total control that night. If I hit him once, I hit him a hundred times. I pushed his face away from me. I'm surprised he didn't have scars from my fingernails. When I had nothing left inside of me, I literally fell to my knees and began to cry hysterically. Joe had sobered up by this time and knelt to the ground and covered my body with his body. I remember being on my knees. I had my face buried in the carpet and I was rocking back and forth. I kept screaming, "I can't take anymore. I can't take anymore!"

Joe knelt over me like a mother who was trying to protect her child from an explosion. I somehow managed to fight my way out of his grip. As I got up, I turned around and hit him as hard as I could with my fist. I ran into the bathroom and got sick. I began to hyperventilate. I was crying so vehemently I could not breathe. Joe tried to calm me down. But everytime he got near me, I took a swing at him and ran into the other room. I ended up in the downstairs bedroom curled up on the daybed.

Joe was crying and kept saying, "I love you."

All I could do was rock back and forth and repeat, "Don't hurt me anymore; **please** don't hurt me anymore!"

Everytime Joe touched me, I gasped and pulled away in complete terror. I kept reciting the same thing

over, "I can't take anymore. Please, don't hurt me anymore." I felt like I was having a nervous breakdown. I
think Joe was convinced I was having one.

After fifteen minutes of begging him not to hurt
me anymore, Joe grabbed me and pulled me next to
him. I fought to loose myself from his grip, but this time
he would not let go. I tried to hit him and get away. He
grabbed my arms and pulled them next to my body as
he pulled my body next to his. He held me next to him
until I quit fighting him. I finally collapsed in his arms and
cried out one last time, "Please, don't hurt me anymore."

Joe and I must have been connected at the very
depths of our being. I will never forget the moment I felt
the disconnection take place. It was such a sobering
feeling. As he continued to hold me, I felt Joe now
rocking back and forth as if he was rocking a baby to
sleep. I looked into his eyes. I saw that he had tears
rolling down his face. He appeared to be in a trance.

"I'm not going to hurt you anymore, Baby. I
promise. I'm not going to hurt you anymore." He kept
repeating that line as he stared into space. He continued to rock me and hold me next to him.

I don't remember anything else about that night
and I don't remember anything about the next morning.
All I remember is Joe was still with me and for the next
two weeks, he was home on time six out of seven nights
of the week. The few nights that he wasn't home on
time, he had been out drinking. He tried to pick fights
and get me to kick him out, but I couldn't do it. It had
just about killed me to go through that once; I couldn't
go through it again. Joe would have to leave me.
Whether it was good, bad, right or wrong, I could never
leave him. And I could never kick him out. If Joe was
going to leave, it was going to have to be his decision
completely.

It was the weekend of August 13, 1989. Joe and I had gone to bed early. He told me that he needed to go out of town the next day, but would be back home on Tuesday night. We got ready for work the next morning and left the house at the same time. We said our goodbyes, gave our goodbye kisses and said our "I love you's".

Although I missed Joe and wanted my marriage to work, I had to admit that it was nice having peace in the house for a change. I took the opportunity to relax and get my thoughts together. I knew that I loved Joe deeply, but I needed a miracle for my marriage to work out. I just did not have it in me to fight anymore.

Tuesday morning, I woke up and trotted down the stairs to let my dog outside. I started to walk through the den toward the french doors that opened to our backyard. I almost had a heart attack as I ran into Joe walking out of the downstairs bedroom. I must have jumped back three feet. I gasped with startlement when I saw him. He had on jeans, no shirt and he was barefoot.

In shock, I asked him, "What are you doing here? I thought you were going out of town."

His reply was simply, "I didn't go."

I asked him, "What time did you get home?" He told me that he had gotten home around 11:00 P.M.

"Joe, I was up at 11:00 P.M."

"No, you weren't," he said, "I came upstairs and you were sprawled out all over the bed sound asleep and the television was on."

I am surprised that I had enough energy or courage to ask my next question. Somehow I knew that the answer was not going to be what I wanted to hear. Joe looked so dissipated as he stood at the bottom of the stairs without his shirt or shoes. He was so incredibly handsome, but on that particular morning - all I could see was a frame. It was as if there were no life on the inside. Joe had already died.

"Where did you go?" I summoned the strength to ask.

I could feel myself turn my emotions off as I prepared for his reply. For the first time in weeks, Joe looked me straight in the eye. He said, "I had a meeting with a broker and then I went to the Texas Bluebonnet Club." He continued to gape as if he were trying to communicate something to me that he could not bring himself to put into words.

I knew Joe had made his decision. As I looked deep into his eyes, my eyes filled with tears. He looked at me with absolutely no emotion. There was no anger, no sadness, no remorse. . . just an empty, expressionless body. I felt the tears roll down my face. They began to drip off of my chin as I looked into his eyes. The lumps in my throat were permeating my passage way where I could not even speak. I swallowed, trying to clear the lump so I could say something, but I didn't know what to say. My knees collapsed underneath me as I fell to the stairs.

Looking up into Joe's anesthetized expression, I said, "It's not going to work. . . is it, Joe?"

He looked at me and with what appeared to be absolutely no feeling. He said, "No. It's not."

I asked the question that all women ask when the man they are in love with is walking out the door. I said, "Joe, you have nothing to lose now, Baby.  You can be honest with me.  Is there someone else?"

He said, "No, there's no one else."

"So, what you're telling me is that you don't love me anymore?"  I was frantically searching for the reason that Joe was walking out of my life.  I knew it had to be something that was wrong with me or that I wasn't good enough.

Joe started to get emotional, which he despised. He wouldn't look at me.  I pleaded for him to answer me. He still wouldn't look at me.  I got in front of him and forcefully turned his face where he could not look away. "Damn it, Joe, you answer me!  Tell me that you don't love me anymore!"

He couldn't do it.  His eyes filled with tears and the truth was written all over his face.  He still loved me. He had never stopped loving me, but Joe could not fight anymore.

"I do love you," he said as his voice cracked. Tears began to fill his eyes.  "It's not that," he continued. "I'm just numb.  I just have to get out of here."

"Joe, just tell me.  What did I do wrong?  If there's not anyone else, then it's got to be that you don't love me anymore.  Just be honest with me.  Joe, you have nothing to lose now. Please, just tell me that you don't love me anymore!"

He couldn't do it.  Everytime that he looked me in the eye, he started to cry.

"I'm just incapable of being married'" he said. "I'm just not good at it."

When he said that, I didn't even care if my marriage stayed together. I just couldn't stand the pain of seeing that look in his eyes; wanting to reach out so desperately, but having given up believing that it was possible for him to work through his pain. I only knew one thing. Joe had felt so unloved in his life. I refused to have him walk out of my life without knowing there was one person on this Earth that believed in him and would always love him.

"I don't buy it, Joe," I screamed. "You have been determined to sabotage this marriage ever since I got sick. You are so damned determined to prove your father right. . . that you're not good enough and that nobody could ever love you. Well, I don't buy it!!! You **are** good enough and I **do** love you!"

"I'm just numb" he said.

"If that's how you feel, then you do need to get out of here." I want your stuff out of here by noon. You can leave the key on the mantle, just lock the bottom lock." I was no longer crying although I felt like my heart had been cut completely out of my body.

I looked at Joe and I saw the man that I was so in love with; the loving, compassionate, sensitive man that was buried deep within this other person.

He again said, with tears in his eyes, "I just need some time. I am just **numb**. I love you, but I'm just not good at marriage."

I was so tired of hearing that. "I'm not crazy about marriage either, Joe. That's why I waited so long to get married. If I didn't desperately want a family, I probably would have never gotten married." I told him.

What Joe said really surprised me. I didn't understand it then and I'm not sure I completely understand his comment now. "Well, good," he said, "Maybe now we can get back to normal."

I questioned what he meant. "Joe, it sounds like you don't want to lose me, but you don't want to be married either. Do you want to date other people? Is there someone else?" I was so confused.

He looked at me as if he were trying to hold on; as if he didn't want to close the door for fear that he would lose me for good. I had told him on many occasions, "I will literally lay down and die for someone that I love. You look up the word commitment in the dictionary and you see my picture. But when it's over - it's over."

Joe said with what appeared to be complete earnestness, "No, I don't want to date anyone else. I want to spend the rest of my life with you, but I just can't be married. God knows you have given me more love and support and freedom than anyone ever could have.

The conversation was getting nowhere. I had to be on the other side of Dallas within thirty minutes. I started to leave. I got in my car and pulled away only to find Joe's image in my rear view mirror. He was standing outside holding my dog in his arms. This time he had a shirt on. He was still barefoot. He watched me drive off until I turned the corner and could no longer see him.

He had been the man that totally changed my life. He had loved me when I felt the most unloved. The man that I was going to grow old with was now gone forever. I didn't know how I was going to live without him.

All the way to work, I cried. I cried about my marriage, but I also cried about Joe. He had made a decision not only about our relationship, but he had also made a decision about himself. I think that's what hurt the most.

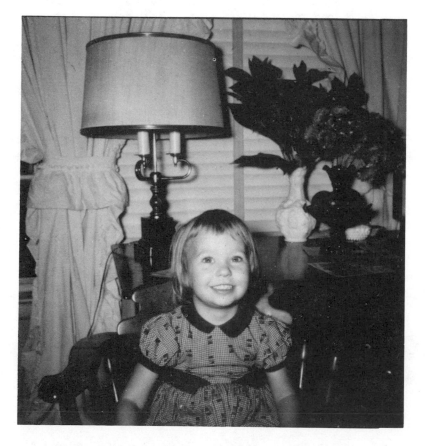

"THANK YOU FOR FIGHTING FOR ME"
Trent P.

Born: 12/27/88
Received Bone Marrow Transplant    07/12/91

# The Child Within
## is dedicated to

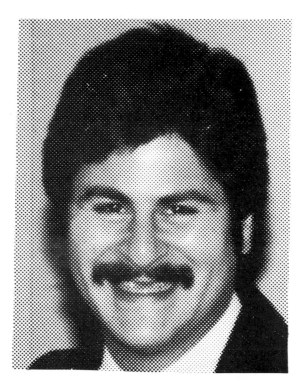

# David Leibs
**who lost his battle to Leukemia
while searching for a donor
Born: October 28, 1956
Died: February 2, 1990**

# PART II

# THE CHILD WITHIN

"David loved the sky and the stars;
flying, and the excitement of space.
Dear Child of our hearts, we hope you
are up there "flying."
We will always love you.  Mom and Dad

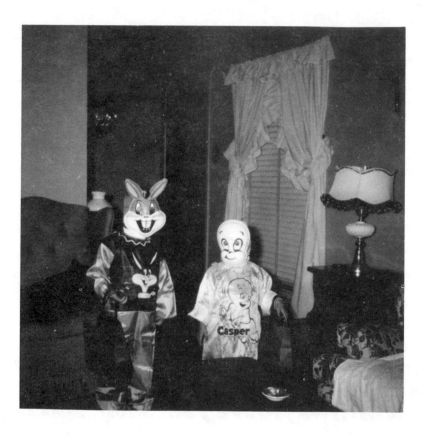

# CHAPTER ONE

## The Decision of a Lifetime

As I always did when I was in deep pain, I began to role play the part I had learned so well as a child. I arrived at work with a smile on my face and a performance that could have won an Academy Award.

The conference was filled with people from various parts of the state. Some I did not know. As I was introducing my self to the new faces I had not met, I would go through my regular routine. I would take a deep breath before I walked up to them, since I was actually so incredibly afraid of them. I would look them straight in the eye, put my shoulders back, put a great big smile on my face, shake their hand and say, "HI! I don't believe I've met you; I'm Christine Mi. . . ." I tried again, "I'm Christine Mich. . ." I could not say my last name without having tears rush to my eyes. All I could think of was how very much I loved Joe and how different my life would be without him. My name wouldn't even be the same. As I thought about the ramifications of what had happened that morning, I knew I had made a big mistake. I had to get home and save my marriage.

It was 8:45 A.M. when I finally stood up to the microphone and welcomed the guests to the conference. I introduced the guest speakers, said my "thank you's" and ran to the car. I called my office to tell them that I would not be back for a few hours.

If the police had been out on patrol that morning, I probably would have been arrested. I drove 80 M.P.H. so I could catch Joe before he moved out. I couldn't let him go. I loved him so much. I needed him. He could do whatever he wanted. I didn't care. I just wanted him with me. I pulled up in front of my house, jumped out of the car and ran to open the door.

"Joe.....", I screamed. I ran through the house looking for him. I opened the door to his closet. That's when I knew I was too late. Joe was gone.

I walked over to the last place I had seen Joe standing. I could still feel his presence. I reached out to touch him. I knew he was gone, but I just wanted to feel his skin next to mine one more time. I remembered the look on his face when I had forced him to look at me just two hours earlier. As I thought about the tears streaming down his face when he said, "I do love you. I'm just numb," I fell to the floor crying. How was I going to live without him? Oh, God, I loved him so much!!

I looked around the house to see what he had taken with him. Just about everything in the house was mine. He had few personal possessions. His console TV was still sitting in the study, along with some of his books. For the most part, everything of his was gone.I realized that it would not be long before Joe would return for the rest of his possessions.

I kept thinking, "How am I going to go on?" I was so afraid. The thought of having to tell everyone that Joe and I were no longer together was more than I could handle. But I was going to face the pain  head-on and I was not going to run from it.

That was a good plan until I thought about making that plan a reality. It meant I would have to face my parents who had been married for 34 years and who saw divorce as the unpardonable sin, along with all of the other sins I had listed under my name. I already felt like a complete failure around them. This just proved their point. Nonetheless, I knew they were going to be the most difficult thing of all to face. I took a deep breath and decided that I would tackle that one first.

I was shaking as I dialed their number. My dad answered the phone. I said, "Dad, Joe left this morning. I'm at home."

I will never forget his words. "Oh, really," he said. "Where did he go. . .to Shreveport?" Here, I was telling my father that my husband had left me and he thought I meant to go on a business trip. When I explained what had happened, Dad said he would be right over. I was sitting on the stairs crying when he arrived.

I told my dad what had been said that morning. "Dad, he had to have a place to go to get out of here so fast. I think he is seeing someone else." My father found that very difficult to believe, but he did agree that Joe had the move planned to happen so fast. He also agreed that it wouldn't be long before Joe would be back for the rest of his possessions.

"He's not going to leave that T.V. here. That's for sure. Maybe I better go before he gets back."

"No, Dad," I screamed. "Please don't leave me. I can't face him alone."

We both looked at each other as we heard a car pull up in the driveway. Joe was back. I had raced home to catch him before he left. Now, I wanted to race out the door before he came in. I sat directly in the same place I had left him a few hours earlier. Now I would have to sit in the same place that he was going to leave me in just a few minutes.

Dad and I sat on the bottom step of my staircase. We watched Joe come through the back gate. He put his key in the lock of the french doors and entered the house. As he got to the breakfast room, he came to a standstill when he saw Dad and I sitting on the stairs.

Joe loved my dad with all his heart. It was tough on both of them to experience an encounter like this. I don't think either one of them realized until that moment that Joe and I breaking up meant their relationship also would end. Joe looked at my dad and then looked at me. Neither of us said a word to him.

As Joe looked down toward the floor my dad said, "Joe, Christine called me and was kind of upset. She asked me to come over." My dad was so diplomatic. He would never think to take anyone's side in their marriage. He respected Joe and believed it was not his place to get involved. He was there to support me; not to berate his son-in-law.    Joe just nodded and stood still.

My heart broke as I looked at Joe's face. I couldn't stand to be in the same room with him. Joe looked at me. I could see the love for me in his eyes. I hated him for what he was doing. I stood up from the bottom step and walked into the downstairs bedroom. Joe followed.

"Why did you tell him?" Joe asked.

I must have looked at him as if he were demented. "What do you mean, why did I tell him?", I asked. "What was I suppose to do . . wait until Thanksgiving and say, 'Gee, I don't know where he is. I guess he went out of town' and then when Christmas comes along say, 'Well, I guess he had other plans'. He was going to find out, Joe. What did you expect me to do?"

"He wants to know what happened," I continued, "and I don't know what to tell him. You go tell him, Joe. Tell him why you're leaving me because I don't even know. You say that you love me; that there's no one else. . . I don't understand. You don't tell someone that you love them and you want to spend the rest of your life with them if you want out of a relationship!"

"I'm just numb." he said.

"Well, then you **do** need to get out of here," I said.

"That's what I'm doing," he said.

I walked over to the bay-window and looked outside. Tears were running down my face. Joe went into the study to pack the rest of his things. I returned to my original position on the stairs next to my dad. We both just sat there and watched Joe pack boxes and carry them to the van he had rented. As Joe was packing, I could see him wiping the tears from his face. Every time Joe carried a box to the van, he would have to walk by Dad and I. We never moved. When he finished moving - he took the key off of his keyring and clenched it in his fist. A tear ran down his face.

"Bye," he said as he bit his lip. He then turned and walked out of the house.

I ran out after Joe. He was sitting in the van gazing into space. He had not started the ignition. He rolled down the window. I said, "Joe, I need to know some things. Are you going to call an attorney?" He looked at me as if I had said something totally absurd. He then looked down at the steering wheel and stared with a great intensity.

After a long period of silence he said, "I want to keep you on my insurance."

"For what?" I asked him. "I have my own insurance. For what, Joe? Until my leukemia comes back or until I **die**?"

"No, not until you **die**," he said.

"Then for what? You can't keep people on your insurance, Joe, when you are divorced," I said in a condescending tone.

"Until you meet someone else or until you decide that you want to get married again," he said as he looked down at the steering wheel.

"**NO WAY, JOE!** You will **NOT** make this my decision. I love you, damn it. I **want** my marriage. This is **your** decision, Joe. You will not make it my responsibility." I screamed. I am sure the neighbors could hear me I was so upset. I was no longer crying. But I was adamant in my determination to let Joe know how I felt. Joe could walk out of my life, but he was going to have to go to his grave knowing that there was nothing that he could do to get me to stop loving him. This was his decision; not mine.

Joe got out of the van. We stood on the back patio and talked. My eyes never left his face. I don't think I even blinked. My expression never changed. After a few minutes, he looked down at the ground. "Maybe something will change," he said as if he had a specific thing in mind. His demeanor dictated that there was more to this story than I knew.

"Like what?" I asked him.

He got very solemn and repeated his comment. "I don't know. Maybe something will change." He looked up at me with the greatest of equanimity. "I don't want a divorce though."

Joe reached out and touched my hand. "I'll call you on Friday," he said.

That was the last time that I ever heard from Joe. He was going out of town the next day on business. Friday arrived. There was no message on my recorder.

He never called me again.    After that day, we never spoke again.

     I thought the best thing for me to do under the circumstances was to go back to work that day.    The first thing I did when I got back to the office was to call the telephone information service to see if Joe had a new number listed.    The telephone company did have a new number listed. It was unpublished.    I called again to make sure I had been given the correct information. There was another Joe Michael that had a new number. It was in the same area of town as the bars that Joe frequented.    I wrote down the address and looked in the phone book.    It was the same apartment complex that Joe had lived in a few years before we met.

     The rest of the day was filled with calling friends and telling them what had happened.    I didn't cry because I was still in shock most of the day.    I made arrangements to meet a friend after work. She had been through a very painful divorce a few years before and was extremely sympathetic. She described the various stages that I would go through during this process.

     On the way to her apartment, there was something inside of me that said, "Go see Ginger."    Ginger was a counselor who worked with our company employee assistance program.    As that thought went through my mind, I looked up and I was two blocks from her office. I decided to go see her. She was so glad to see me.

     "Hi!" I said with my normal great big smile.  "You know any good counselors?"

     As she reached out to give me a hug and a smile, she said, "Well, I'm a good counselor."  I began to cry.

"Christine, what's the matter?    Come into my office," she said.  I put my head on her desk and continued to cry.

I looked up and said, "My husband left me this morning.  Ginger, I am so in love with him.  I don't know what I'm going to do.  I feel like calling my doctor and telling him to put me back in the hospital.  I can't go through this."

As all "good counselors" do, she said, "Christine, tell me what happened.  Do you know?"

I talked about Joe's anger at not finding a job for an extended time period, about his mother's suicide, about his anger with me for being sick.  I talked to her about him coming in late and about the fights we had.

"Ginger, I think he's seeing someone else," I said.

"Oh, Christine, you wish he were seeing someone else.  That would be easy for you to handle.    At least, with that.. you could compete."

She looked at me and waited for me to draw my own conclusions from the comment she made.  I looked at her and then looked down.  Ginger knew I was in denial.  I had not mentioned anything about Joe's drinking.

"Let me ask you something," Ginger said, "Does Joe drink?"

I said, "Well, yeah, I mean...once in a while he'll have a couple of beers.  But he never orders anything when we go out and we don't keep alcohol in the house."

"What is he like when he drinks?" she asked.

As we talked about the disease of alcoholism, I asked her, "When does someone who drinks that has problems become a 'problem drinker?'" I was doing everything to keep from admitting that Joe was sick.

Ginger answered with a reply that I will never forget. She said, "When it becomes a problem, Christine." Although I worked with chemical dependency, it was as if someone had siphoned the knowledge from my brain. No matter what I knew about the disease of addiction, it did not apply to my present life. Yet, I knew it was the truth. That was the first time I admitted Joe was an alcoholic. I had called him everything except what he really was. I had called him "a high risk candidate." I called him insensitive for not calling me when he was going to be late, but I had never been able to acknowledge that Joe was an alcoholic. Somehow I thought if I could just love him enough. . . if I could just prove to him that he was a wonderful, loving, caring, talented man - then things would be okay. He wouldn't "turn into" an alcoholic. The problem was I was too late. I just didn't know how late.

Ginger helped me a lot that first day. She talked to me about the need to take care of myself. She suggested that since alcoholism is a "family disease," I get into some counseling quickly. "Christine, after what you've been through, it is imperative that you take care of yourself. You need to go to counseling and take care of **YOU**. Get plenty of rest and exercise." She gave me a list of people to contact. "I also think that you need to get into a group. Since you don't know what is going to happen, Al-a-non would be a big help to you," she said. I left her office feeling much better for having stopped to see her. I had a plan of action.

My friend, Ann, was waiting for me when I got to her apartment. I told her about Ginger's diagnosis of Joe's alcoholism. She said, "Christine, you know I think she's right. My brother is an alcoholic and that's exactly the way he acted with his wife. I mean so did Mark, (her ex-husband), but he was just crazy." We both laughed. It felt so good to laugh for the first time all day.

We went out to eat that night. Although neither of us drink, we ordered a pitcher of beer with our meal. Before the evening was over, I was pretty tipsy. I remember telling her, "You know, I think I could handle this if I just stayed in a bar every night. No wonder Joe does this."

After dinner, we decided to drive around. I just happened to have the address with me that I had gotten from the telephone operator. Joe's apartment was only a few blocks from Ann's apartment. As we drove through the apartment complex, I crouched down in the seat and peeked over the dashboard. I had no idea where Joe's apartment was. The last thing I wanted was for him to see me driving by looking for him. As we drove through each parking lot, Ann would look for Joe's car while I hid. When we found his car in the parking lot, I felt my heart melt. All I could feel for him was love.

I had found Joe. At least now I knew where he was. I picked up my car at Ann's apartment and drove back by Joe's apartment. As I looked up at the four windows, I wondered which room was his. Was he asleep? Then. . . a tinge of pain came upon me. Was he by himself? So many thoughts were going through my mind. As I was driving home, it dawned on me that it was *that* morning that Joe moved out. He already had a phone. He already had an apartment. He had the whole thing planned. I drove home and cried myself to sleep.

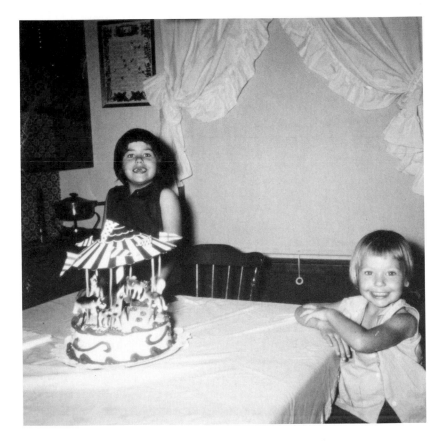

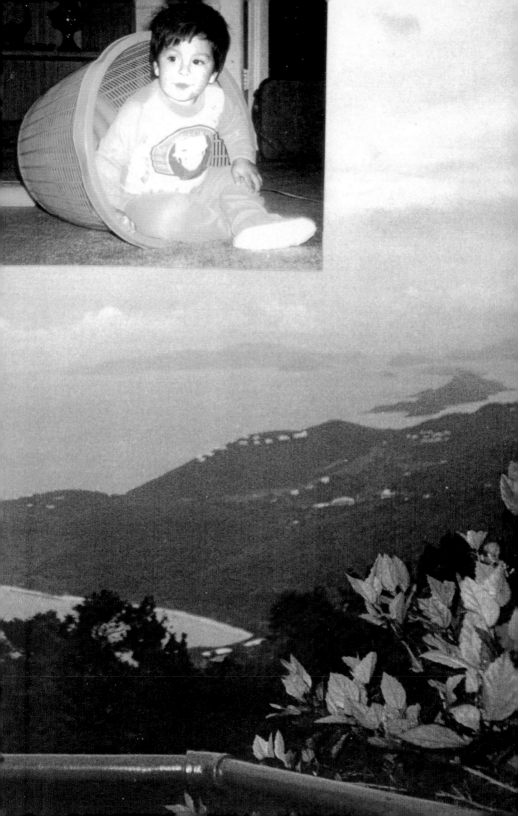

# CHAPTER TWO

## You've Got to take Care of Yourself

Sleeping that first night without Joe was not that difficult. Since he traveled three days a week, I had become fairly use to it. I knew the difficult time would be on the weekend. Friday nights were always our night out to eat. We would usually go to some nice restaurant, get a steak, come home and watch TV and make love for hours. I knew that getting through the first weekend without him was going to be the toughest.

I made an appointment for Saturday morning with Steve - a counselor who had worked for me the previous year. We had become good friends. He was in Adult Children of Alcoholics. I talked with him about going to Al-A-non with me. He was more than willing. He said, "I don't go a lot anymore, but I'd love to go. Which group did you want to go to?"

I had no idea. I was a professional in the field. I told other people where to go counseling. I had a list, but I didn't know which group was good. One thing I am very thankful for is that I have a lot of resources - I have many friends in the profession who are therapists and work with recovery. After making a phone call, I found out the best Al-A-non group. The following evening, Steve met me at that location. We got there early so we could talk. He said, "Christine, this is Joe's problem. There is nothing you can do about it. You have got to take care of yourself."

I thought I was taking care of myself. I made an appointment for counseling. I was about to go to my first Al-A-non meeting. A friend of mine had agreed to work out with me at the health club every night. What else was I suppose to be doing?

The time came for the meeting to start. Steve and I went inside and sat down at a table filled with strange faces. Everyone introduced themselves. I felt a little strange. I knew how 12-step programs worked. But still, when it was my turn to introduce myself and everyone simultaneously said, "Hi, Christine," I somehow felt that I was the one who was the alcoholic.

I decided to "tough it out." When it was my turn to share, I told the story of what just happened in my life. My "toughing it out" lasted about 30 seconds into my sharing. I burst into tears. Suddenly, it was as if the whole room were attacking me. Everyone was talking to me at the same time. They all jumped to my rescue, handed tissues to me and said, "This is your first time - isn't it?" They told me about a new-comers group that I might want to attend first. Everyone was touching me and saying, "It's okay to hurt. It's okay to be angry". . . and then that same statement that I was getting pretty tired of hearing. . . "Christine, you've got to take care of yourself."

Never in my life could I show anger or pain in front of someone that I was not extremely close to. I would usually cover it up by saying, "That's okay" and smiling. That way they would still accept me and still love me. For the first time, I didn't care if these people loved me because I hated them.

"My God, he just left," I said. "I feel like everyone here is jumping down my throat." I don't remember what else I said, but I knew that whoever told me that was the best group in town should have their license revoked. I was **NOT** going back there.

Steve and I talked afterward. "Christine, I think you were really a little tough on those people. They weren't jumping down your throat."

"Steve, he's been gone two days. Everybody I talk to keeps saying that I need to take care of myself. I feel like I did when I was little. I can't even do that right. I don't understand what people expect me to do", I screamed. Steve and I talked for an hour and then I left to go home.

I sat outside on my deck and thought about the evening. I thought about my entire life. It was as if I was speaking a different language than everyone else. I could not understand what people were saying to me. I just wanted someone to tell me what I was "suppose" to do. I would do what they said. I would do **anything**. I had always been willing to do what other people said. I just didn't want to hurt anymore. I wanted the pain to go away. As I was looking up at the stars, I thought about God and how much I loved Him. I always said that He made my life complete. But I was still searching. If I were really honest with myself, I wasn't sure that God had really ever made me happy. I would never be able to admit that to myself or especially to anyone else.

I had my "wild days," but since college. . . God was my life. I "walked the walk, I talked the talk." Everyone thought I was so "spiritual." I thought about the way that I was introduced so often: "This is the most Godly woman I've ever met. You'll just love getting to know her. She really walks with the Lord." As I thought about those comments it made me sick to my stomach. Everyone thought I was so awesome, but NONE of them really knew me.

And then I thought about Joe. He was the only one who really knew me. What a mountain top! I strive all of my life to be able to <u>really</u> open up and share my inner self with someone. I finally arrive after a life of insecurity and fear and the one person that showed me the path. . . just pushed off the top.

"God, I have got to learn to love myself," I cried out. Tears began to run down my face. "Lord, I am so afraid. I don't know how to live without being "perfect." The only person that I wasn't "perfect" for left me. I can't live without him, God. Oh, Jesus. . . teach me to love myself. God, I'm going to die. I can feel it. God, help me," I cried.

I went inside and laid on the floor and wept. My dog came up and started to lick my face. "Valentine, I miss your daddy." As I made that comment, Valentine perked up his ears, looked out the window and ran to the door. He knew "Daddy" meant Joe. As I watched my dog whining for Joe to open the door so he could greet him, I buried my face in the carpet. And the next day was supposed to be the toughest.

To keep my mind off Joe, I decided to start working on my doctorate again. Classes were starting the following week. I would have to hurry in order to get accepted and begin on time. I thought that it would be good therapy for me. Since I was working on my doctorate in Human Resource Development, I decided it would be a great time to take the course entitled "Chemical Dependency Counseling." It was a required course for me and after all, they were offering the class at the local extension center close to my house. During lunchtime, I went to the extension school of the university to pick up the forms that I needed. As I was driving back to the office, I had this overpowering need to drive by Joe's apartment. It was the first time that I ever felt so out of control. I felt if I did not drive by, I would not make it through the day. I thought, "This must be what an alcoholic feels like when he has to have a drink." I became obsessed with finding out if Joe was back in town and if he was even working.

When I arrived at this apartment complex, there were maintenance personnel all around Joe's building. I realized that I would not be able to pursue my investi-

gation during the day. I returned to my office. At 4:30
P.M., I drove by Joe's apartment complex one more
time. His car was there. I went home and waited for Joe
to call. The phone never rang. There was no message
on my recorder.    I kept staring at the phone and
remembering his last words, "I'll call you on Friday."

Friday had arrived. . . the day I had waited for all
week.   As the time progressed, I became more depressed.  I don't know why I thought Joe really meant it
when he said he would call. It wasn't any different than
it was before he moved out. I made four trips back and
forth from my house to Joe's apartment juggling the
tasks of checking my answering machine and trying to
find out more information about Joe. The pursuit was
only causing me to become more frustrated and depressed. I finally decided that Joe was **not** going to call
me; he probably never would.

I tried desperately to accept that fact, but I could
not let go. I drove the twenty miles back to Joe's apartment. I pulled into the apartment complex next to his,
parked my car under a tree and sat and waited. I kept
telling myself, "Christine, if you can just get through this
night, you won't ever have to do this again. You will have
*made* it through your first Friday night without him."
At 12:01 A.M., I looked at the clock in my car and said,
"I made it." Joe was still not home, he had not called
me, but at least it wasn't Friday anymore.

The following week was Joe's birthday.  I went
shopping to help pass the time away. I found myself
picking up polo shirts and golf shirts for Joe, only to put
them back down. I realized I was going to have to give
him the time that he needed. I decided there would be
no harm in sending him a birthday card. Joe didn't have
a lot of friends and I was sure his birthday would not be
a happy one. I chose a special card and wrote a note
letting Joe know how very much I loved him.

I continued to go to counseling and went to Al-A-non everyday.  I spent most of my work hours touring new treatment facilities for the employee assistance program.  I made it a point to talk to the "addiction-ologist" about Joe.  In each case, I would hear the same thing.  "Christine," they would say, "You act as though this is your problem.  You really do need to take care of yourself.  Until Joe 'hits bottom', he's not going to come home.  He's got to want to stop drinking."

I heard what they were saying.  I knew I could not let Joe back in the house unless he was in a treat-ment program.   But how was he going to get into a treatment program?   Joe probably would die first and I couldn't stand to watch him die.  Just in case he did "bottom out", which I felt sure would be in only a few weeks, I had him pre-admitted to two residential chemi-cal dependency programs.  I also got it cleared through his insurance company so all I would have to do is take him to the hospital.  I continued to be obsessed with what Joe was doing.  I kept telling myself that within weeks he would "bottom out," get into treatment, we would get back together and live happily ever after.  Each night that I wasn't in class, I would drive by his apartment and park two parking lots away.  I would sneak through his apartment complex, make sure he wasn't home, and slip in through the same unlocked door on his patio.

I took inventory of how much liquor he had consumed.  I would review his bills and his checkbook to see how much he was spending.  Within one month from the first time I entered his apartment, Joe was spending an additional $1500.00 a month in liquor and bar tabs.  He was going through approximately $600.00 undesignated cash a week.  I didn't understand where the money was coming from.  Joe made good money, but his salary was not enough to be spending that amount on luxury items.  He still had to pay rent and child support.

On one occasion I went so far as to rent a car for the weekend. I put a scarf on my head. I knew Joe would not recognize me. I was no longer wearing my wig. I punched out the lenses of my sunglasses, dressed in black and entered his apartment. I had been listening to Joe's messages when one night my heart almost quit beating. Most of his messages were from business associates trying to find him. A couple of men had apparently become Joe's drinking buddies. They were always intoxicated when they called. This particular night I heard a voice I had not heard before. It was a man with a very deep voice and a Hispanic accent.

"Joe, this is Jesse Gonzales," the voice said, "You did a little job for me about six weeks ago. I heard you were interested in making some extra money. Give me a call. I have another little job for you to run." I stared at the recorder for at least ten minutes without moving until I finally remembered where I was. I knew that Joe could be coming home any minute. He usually got home around 1:00 A.M. I knew because I sat in the parking lot next to his apartment complex waiting for him to come home almost every night.

After hearing the message that sounded so much like a drug deal, I became even more obsessed with finding out the truth. I searched every inch of his apartment for any type of drug paraphernalia I could find. I then remembered the trips to the convenience store that Joe made every morning to get a diet coke. He would NEVER let me go with him. It was only one block from our house. I thought about the time at Thanksgiving that we got into the big fight concerning my going to the store with him. Many things were starting to make sense. They made sense for someone else's life though. I continued to search for some other answer. Surely Joe couldn't be doing drugs. It would explain the mood swings, the amount of money he was spending, but my God. . running drugs?

I talked to several people in the field of chemical dependency recovery and to people that I knew were active users. I could not find one person to disagree with me. Every one of them said, "Christine, Joe is delivering drugs." If he ever went out of town, he went to Houston and to the port cities of Louisiana. I was told those two places are the biggest drug markets in the south for picking up deliveries. I knew several under-cover drug investigators. They told me that Joe was apparently not only using, but delivering cocaine on his business trips.

This was the man that I prayed with and the man that I went to church with. This was the man that had rededicated his life to the Lord just a few months before his mother had committed suicide. As I continued to search for answers, I found out Joe had been using and selling cocaine when we met. Working in Human Resources, I knew the people who were in treatment, so I started using them as "sources."

Joe had been fired from his job with our company. It was supposedly for stealing some sand that amounted to $4.20. He was in management and his supervisor, who was a close friend of his, said he just could not let that happen when Joe was in a leadership position as he was. We had an undercover drug investigation shortly after Joe got fired. Many of Joe's employees were terminated for drug possession. I contacted some of those people and found out Joe was handing out packages of cocaine to his employees the night we announced our engagement. The more investigating I did, the more devastated I became. Joe had not called me and he was not making any attempt to put closure on the marriage.

I was in total darkness. I didn't know from one day to the next if I was going to be married, if Joe was taking time to get his life together or if he was just avoiding the entire issue. All I knew was that my husband was dying and there was nothing I could do about it. Members of my church were calling Joe and leaving messages on his recorder. "Joe, we love you and we miss you. If there's anything we can do or if you just want to talk, call anytime," they would say. Joe would never return their phone calls.

There was one person that he would talk to. It was one of my closest friends. She wrote him once a week. She never put pressure on him. She told him that she was praying for him and she missed seeing him at church. During one of their conversations, she told him, "Joe, you need to let Christine know something. She's in limbo. There is nothing worse than just not knowing. If you would just let her know what your plans are. Joe, Christine loves you. I think the way she puts it is that she is 'head over heels in love with you'." He told Debra that the lifestyle that he was living would destroy me. "Debra," he said, "she couldn't live through the lifestyle that I'm living right now. I know Christine. It would kill her."

I was getting to the point I could not stand the pain any longer. I had become total dysfunctional at work. I was making a 4.0 in my graduate course, but it was only because I was trying to learn more about chemical dependency. Half of my subject and interpretation papers were about Joe. I felt as though I did not fit in anywhere. I couldn't go back to our couples class, although they never quit reaching out to me. I visited the single's department at my church and I knew I did not belong there. I still had Joe's last name. What was I doing in a singles group?

My counseling sessions were helping, but Al-A-Non was my savior. It was the only thing in my life that was helping me to learn to take care of myself. It took me several weeks to realize I was not there to learn how to fix Joe. I thought after that discovery, I knew the real reason for Al-a-Non: it was to learn how to live with your alcoholic. It took a few more months before I finally started to understand what people had been trying to tell me all along. When they said, "Christine, you have got to take care of yourself" - they knew Joe was not the only one with a problem.

I soon discovered I was also an addict. As much as Joe was addicted to drugs, I was addicted to him. Al-a-non was not a support group for those women trying to hold on to their husbands. It was a support group for those people trying to learn how to take care of themselves; no matter what the outcome. I looked back on the events of my life: the patterns were there.

Everything I encountered in life was an obsession. I had almost been an alcoholic during college. When I stopped drinking, I became a work-a-holic. Then. . .a religious fanatic. . .and now a love addict.

I still struggled with the concept of focusing on myself. It was contrary to everything I had been taught. All my rewards came from taking care of everyone else. It never occurred to me that I was the one that needed help. I didn't understand what it all meant. I spent my life searching for something that would make me complete. I thought I had found that with Joe and my baby. They fulfilled the deepest desires of my heart.

I knew Joe had to fix himself. I couldn't do it for him. I had enough to handle in taking care of myself. I had to get free of my own addiction. The thought of doing that terrified me. I had no idea how to let go. I knew that somewhere there was an answer for me. . . if I only knew where to look.

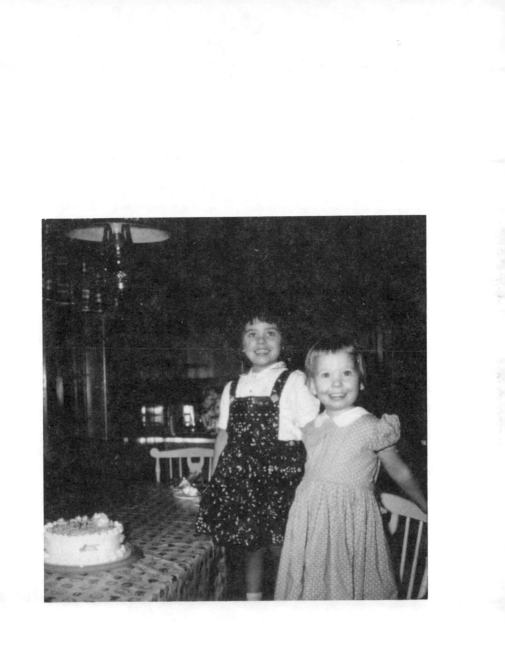

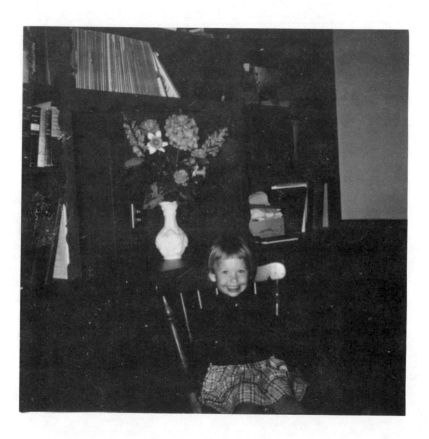

# CHAPTER THREE

## *God Grant Me the Serenity*

I think the thing that helped me the most about attending a twelve-step program is that for the first time in my life I did not have anyone's expectations by which I was having to live. I have always been my own worse critic. No matter what I did, I made sure it was a success. Everywhere I went, I played a different role.

If the goal was to reach the height of "spiritualism," I made sure everyone around me thought that I was the most "godly" woman alive. If the goal was to be creative, I would stay up for hours developing new programs. I could be whatever anyone wanted me to be. I had learned to role play whatever was needed for any given situation.

As I walked through each of the "twelve steps" with my fellow "Al-a-nons", I was challenged with a new role - that of being the perfect addict.

The steps were easy to remember. They were posted everywhere you looked. The first step, "We admitted we were powerless over alcohol-that our lives had become unmanageable". . .that step was easy for me. There was no question whether Joe's life was unmanageable. His life being in chaos made my life unmanageable. I could accept that. It was weeks later before I realized nobody was talking about Joe's life. It was MY life that had become unmanageable. The truth was I had always known that my life was unmanageable. My problem was I just couldn't let anyone else know my life was unmanageable.

Step Two was also a given. It read, "Came to believe that a Power greater than ourselves can restore us to sanity." Being raised in a family where my father was a deacon in a Southern Baptist Church, that step was not open for discussion. I was never allowed to question whether there was a Power greater than myself that could restore me to sanity. . . I was never allowed to be "insane." _Those_ things were never discussed.   If I admitted I had faults and I struggled, then Jesus wouldn't love me. With those two steps being a "given,"  I went immediately for Step Three.

"Made a Decision to turn our will and our lives over to the care of God as we understand him. That is the part that I struggled with. "Made a decision to turn our will and our lives over to the care of God *as we understood Him.*" I had seen the hand of God in my life so many times. I prayed to Him daily. I saw Him perform miracles in my life. How could I now be questioning my understanding  of God?

I thought about the night I sat on my deck a couple of months earlier. I remember thinking "I'm not sure God has ever made me happy." I was so afraid to even ponder that thought.   My faith had gotten me through my life. I loved Jesus with all my heart. When I had enough courage to take a quick peek inside, I don't think He really ever made me happy though. Turning my will and my life over to Him was easy. But I was starting to wonder. . . did Jesus really love me? Did He love me for *no* reason. . . not for what I *did* or for the *type of person* I was, but. . .just because He loved me?

I never felt there was any person in my life who really did love me . My grandfather was the *only* person. There were people in my life who **wanted** me.   They wanted me to be their friend because I was fun to be with or because I listened to their problems until all hours of the night. They wanted to marry me because I was always loving and encouraging.   They wanted to hire me because I did such a wonderful job. Everyone wanted something.   But I didn't know anyone that

wanted me *just for me.* I thought the exception had
been Joe. But I was wrong. I didn't understand anything
that was happening in my life. I knew that God was my
Higher Power and He was the answer. I just didn't know
what He looked like anymore.

Praying the <u>Serenity Prayer</u> helped a lot. I would
pray:

***God grant me the serenity***
***to accept the things I cannot change,***
***the courage to change the things I can***
***And the wisdom to know the difference***

I found that I didn't have to understand what or
who God was. I just had to believe. I held on to that
belief much like a person who has been blind from birth
must hold on to the belief that they are not going to fall
through the earth. A blind person doesn't know what
the sky or earth looks like, but he somehow knows that
he is steady and that is enough. That is how I related to
God at that point in my life.

Working through some pain in my own life only
brought up more pain. As I learned more about myself,
I discovered there was more to uncover. At times it
seemed impossible that I would ever get through the
years of self doubt. I had no answers. I didn't even
know what the questions were. My purpose had been
living my life for everyone else. Now I had to find **something** to fill that void within myself.

I was petrified that Joe was going to be killed
during one of his drug runs. I tried to let go. No matter
how much I tried, I could not walk away. I kept picturing
Joe lying in the street bleeding. I couldn't walk away
from him. My vows were the most sacred thing in my life.
I had taken them "until death do us part". I was convinced if they were broken, then one of us was sup-

posed to be dead. Joe stayed by my side while I close to death. I couldn't walk away from him now. His disease was not any different than my having leukemia.

During the weeks following my discovery of Joe's addiction, I began to see bruises on my legs. After having leukemia once, I knew those bruises were symptomatic, but I didn't even want to think about the possibility of a relapse. Every day a new bruise would appear. I would try to ignore it and say, "Christine, you just hit the machine while you were working out." Each morning my gums would bleed, but I would ignore that, too.

My thoughts were only on Joe; not myself. One night I was driving home from a meeting. I had driven by Joe's apartment on the way. I wasn't thinking about anything in particular. It had become routine to check on Joe. My thoughts were no longer consumed with him although he was always in the back of my mind. As I was driving down the freeway, I heard this voice say, "It's time." Tears rushed to my eyes. I knew that voice. It was the same voice that spoke to me in the hospital the night I was diagnosed. I didn't have to question what the comment meant. I **knew** God was telling me it was time to let go.

"God, I can't do it.", I said. I was crying so intensely I could barely see the road. Once again I heard the same voice. It said, "Christine, it's time to let go."

I pulled into my driveway and got out of my car. I entered my house and looked at the things Joe had left there. Joe had things that were so precious to him that he had never come to get. I walked into the study. I could feel the presence of God in my house. I wanted to hide from Him. I wanted Him to leave. I knew He was asking me to do something that was going to absolutely destroy me. I walked into the bathroom and looked at myself in the mirror. I had mascara all over my face from tears. My eyes were red and swollen from crying. Wherever I went in my house, the presence of God went with me. It wasn't a peaceful, joyful presence. It felt like a father who was refusing his child's request to play in the street.

I walked back into the study and reached up to get Joe's highschool yearbook from the shelf. I had read it several times. Everyone loved Joe, or "Joey" as he was called in high school. Whenever I started to give up on ever getting through Joe's thick wall of pain, I would pull out his annual and read about the Joey that I knew; the one I sat with under the moonlight. We would talk for hours when we were dating. That is the Joey that I fell in love with. That is the Joey that I married.

My heart broke as I read the inscription in his annual:

*Dear Joey (alias Ben Casey)*
*I sure am glad I'm getting to sign in your annual, because maybe by me telling you on paper how much I think of you, you might remember it. Joey, I hope you know how much I really think of you. I'm afraid I will never equal you in your wonderful faith and belief in God. I really want to thank you for the wonderful talks you've given me, Joey. I just hope one of these days I'll be as informed as you are about the Bible. Honest, Joey, that's the most wonderful thing about you - you're cute, sweet, and most handsome and very popular but you're not like all of the other popular and cute guys. You've got a special shine and glow that comes from knowing the Lord. You not only know Him, but you try to get everyone else to know Him. Joey, your life has already been richly blessed, but hold your horses, pardner, because it's only just begun. You are a won-*

*derful Christian example to all of the students at Pine Branch who love and admire you. I hope that I can be a good of a student to you as you have been a teacher to me.*

*Joey, I hope you come over this summer and give me lessons in life, because so far. . I have learned so many wonderful things from you I know that you are going to make a wonderful doctor and you will bring light to everyone you know. You have a special place in Heaven.*

I closed the annual and began to cry. That stern presence was still in my house. I could feel God waiting for my decision. "I can't do it, God. I love him. I can't let Him die."

As I was crying and thinking about Joe, I saw a picture of him in my mind. He was lying in the street bleeding. He had been shot. He was drunk and reeked with the smell of alcohol. He was high from cocaine and pot. He looked as though he had not shaved in months. I looked into Joe's eyes. Once again, I heard God say "Christine, you've got to let go. . For the first time I realized - I was preventing Joe from falling. We were so connected that somehow Joe knew I would always be there for him. I loved Joe so much and had so much faith in him and in God - that my prayers alone were keeping him from falling. He would have to have no one or nowhere to turn before he would reach out for help.

As long as he didn't have to feel the pain. . . he would survive. In actuality, his protection was killing him just as mine was killing me. I knew what I had to do. I just didn't know if I had the strength to do it.

Throughout my life I tried to live the way I thought Jesus would want me to live. I was constantly striving to give, to love, to forgive. . . and to be that "perfect" little girl so Jesus would love me. I tried to live my life according to the Bible. As I thought about the seriousness of what God was asking me to do, a verse in the book of <u>John</u> came to mind. It reads: "This is my commandment, that you love one another, as I have loved you. Greater love has no one than the man that lays down his life for his brother."

As I was meditating on that verse, a question entered my mind. The question was, "Christine, if you **knew** that by dying tonight and giving up your life you could come back to Earth and be a guardian angel for Joe 24 hours a day. . . if you **knew** that Joe would eventually work through his pain, quit taking drugs and be happy the remainder of his days on this Earth, would you give up your life for him?"

I didn't even have to think about the answer. I would do anything for Joe to be happy; even if it meant dying. As soon as I replied to the question that was presented to me, I felt a heaviness in my heart. I immediately knew that I had given the *wrong* answer. The presence I had felt so strongly in my house was now still and quiet. It was as if God were no longer waiting for my answer. I had made my decision. In reality, I had made my decision before Joe ever left.

I thought about that scenario a long time. Another question was brought to mind. "If you **knew** it was God's will for you to die tonight, would you give up your life for God?" Many times while I was sick and close to death I said, "I don't care if it is **God's** will, I'm not going!" I would always say, "I'm head over heels in love with my husband and I'm expecting my first baby and I'm not going anywhere." I knew what God was trying to tell me. Joe had become my god.

I realized that night that no one should be placed in that position except for God Himself. I had made Joe my god and I expected to be his. I was literally willing to die for Joe in order that he could have a lifestyle that he wanted no part of. I was constantly "laying down my life for my brother" and getting abused because I thought that was God's will for my life. If I failed, I thought that I deserved the pain. It was because I had not been "good enough." At the bottom of all of the pain lived a little girl who didn't believe she deserved to live.

I thought about the verse that says, "Love your neighbor as yourself." I had always loved my neighbor **Instead** of myself. I wanted to make everyone else happy, at my own expense. I knew I was receiving some inner healing concerning my own life. The revelation was so contrary to everything I had been taught. My responsibility was for my own life, "to take care of Christine." It was the comment that everyone had been telling me for months. That was the root of my problem.

I never wanted to look out for myself. I always thought that was a sin. I thought about Al-A-non. . .Step Four: "I made a searching and fearless moral inventory of myself." My God, how was I going to do that? I always talked about how easy it was to complete that step. I never understood why people would agonize over that step with tears. Now it was time for me to work that step. I couldn't even get started.

I thought about my strengths and weaknesses, I could not list one thing that I did well. I could list several things I did not do well. Each time something crossed my mind that could possibly be a strength, I realized it was because Joe thought that I did it well. It wasn't because I believed it myself. Something else would come to mind and it was because my supervisor thought I did it well. It didn't take long to realize that I, Christine, took everyone else's inventory of me. I didn't have an inventory of myself. My entire self esteem was based on what **other** people thought about me. Without other peoples perceptions, I didn't have a self concept.

"Christine, you've got to take care of yourself" -
Those words kept coming to my mind. For the first time
I understood what that meant. As I was deep in thought,
I felt the presence of God return. "Christine, it's time."
The same voice that had spoken to me while I was
driving home was now speaking again. The message
was the same. I had to take care of myself.

As I got up from the chair in my office, I felt a
pain deep within me. My teeth chattered as I attempted
to hold back the tears. I had cried so much in the past
few months. I didn't want to cry anymore. I walked to
the bathroom and looked in the mirror. My arms were
covered with bruises. With a sigh I thought to myself,
"It's not going to do any good, is it God? I'm willing to
die; I'm willing to lay down my life for Joe and it's not
going to do a damn bit of good. I can't save him. I
can't even help him." I mentally saw the same image of
Joe once again. This time I was standing over him and
Jesus was in the background.

I visualized looking into Joe's eyes. I knew I
would have to be the one to end this madness. Joe
would never do it. As I thought about breaking my vows
and walking away from him, I fell to the floor and began
to cry. How was I going to let go of the only thing that
made my life complete? I had reached a point that if
Joe filed for divorce, than I could agree to it. But for me
to be the one to take action for dissolving our marriage
went against everything I believed in. It was impossible
for me to turn my back on someone. . . anyone that was
in pain.

I kept hearing the same words repeated in my
mind: "Greater love has noone than the one who lays
down his life for his brother." That still small voice then
spoke. "Christine, I will never leave you, nor forsake
you. You've got to let go."

I thought laying down my life meant being willing to die for someone.  That would have been easy.  God had never asked me to lose my life for anyone; he merely asked me to lay it down - to give up my own expectations and allow "my brother" the freedom and the dignity to choose his own path to freedom.  He must choose his own journey - for in each journey is where we encounter our oneness.  God made me and has a wonderful plan for my life, but I had to choose to receive it.  I had to choose to go on in order to see the full picture, but I would have to go on without Joe.

When I finally made my decision to "lay down my life," I had no idea how I was going to do it.  I just knew I had to get through it.  I decided to try something I had used when counseling others.  It seemed to be quite helpful.  It was a Gestalt exercise.  Many counselors call it "the empty chair."  It is a wonderful tool for resolving relationship conflicts where the person is no longer available to communicate with the client.  In this case, I was the client.  I wasn't sure who the counselor was.  This "presence" in my house seemed to be playing the part pretty well.

I knew that in order to make this work, I would have to face myself.  I would have to look at myself in the mirror.  I placed Joe's picture on the bathroom cabinet, and I made sure I could see the reflection of myself looking into his eyes.  His eyes were not the eyes I had seen in my mind as I visualized Joe lying in the street.  They were the eyes of Joey.  He looked so different.  I took a deep breath, stood Joe's picture up and looked straight into his eyes.  I was paralyzed with pain.  I wanted so much to call him and have him come home.  I wanted to make love to him the way we always did after a fight.

"Oh, Dear God, my heart. . . .," I cried.  The emotional pain was enough to kill me.  I cried hysterical-ly.  I could feel my body being pushed to its limits to accommodate the needs of my soul. Surely there was another way I could get through this than having to break my vows. I looked in the mirror and was brought back to reality. I once again saw the bruises.

"You're going to die, Christine," I thought. "Not only are you going to die, you are going to kill Joe when you go. You have **got** to let him go. He knows that you love him. He knows that you will always be there for him."

"But, I'm not being there for him," I cried. "I'm turning my back on him."

The battle within myself went on for what seemed like hours. I held Joe's picture in my arms and looked into his eyes. I could feel the incredible passion that I had for him. I could remember the feelings I felt for him when we got married. I thought about the first time that we made love. I remembered the look on Joe's face the first time we heard the baby's heartbeat. I would not allow myself to take my eyes off of his eyes. I began to repeat my marriage vows.

"I, Christine, take you, Joe to be my lawful wedded husband. . . " I could barely breathe I was crying so intensely. My vision was blurred from having my eyes so filled with tears.

"I promise to love, honor and cherish you. . . "

"Oh, God, please don't make me do this. I can't do this. I love him," I screamed. I made myself start from the beginning each time I repressed the pain.

"I, Christine, take you Joe. . . " My very soul was being ripped out.

"In sickness and in health. . . " I could not get past that point without falling apart. Oh, Dear God, what

happened to my marriage?" I screamed. All I could think
about was how Joe never left my side the day we
delivered the baby. He sat by me with tears in his eyes
and never let go of my hand. He kept repeating, "I love
you. I'm right here."

"For richer; for poorer. . ." I had so many memories of conversations with Joe about his unemployment.
He would often say, "I feel like you are the only person
who has ever believed in me. You really do think I'm
good."

I laid on the floor and wailed for an hour before
I could catch my breath and continue. I finally repeated
my vows without taking my eyes off of Joe's picture and
without having to stop in the middle of the process. It
was three hours later when I finally said: **"Until death do
us part."**

I was no longer crying. I put his picture face
down on the bathroom cabinet and looked in the mirror.
I stared into the image of not just what Joe had become,
but what I had become. I could see our entire marriage
right before my eyes. I could see Joe's past and I could
see my past. As I looked into my own reflection, I saw
the image of Joe lying in the street bleeding. He was
inside of me.

I continued. "And, Joe. . . knowing where you
are in your addiction, I choose as an act of **my** will to
step over you. . . ." I saw Joe look up at me from his
drug induced stupor. "**I choose** to step over you, to turn
my back. . . and to walk away. I **willingly** choose to
break my vows and let you go." As I said the last statement, I fell on my knees and wept until early morning.
An authentic sting took place when I released Joe. A
part of me was now gone. Joe was free to go on with his
life however he chose to live it. So was I.

I turned off the light in the bathroom and started to climb the stairs to go to my bedroom. As I walked up the stairs, it was as though I was in a foreign land. Nothing felt familiar. I knew no one and no one knew me. I then realized what I had gone through was not releasing Joe. It was releasing myself, even though I didn't know who "myself" was. I didn't have a choice whether to release Joe. He had made that decision.

I wanted so much to turn my back and walk away, but I was stuck. I had started a process that I knew was going to change my life. I had no idea where or how I would find the answers, but at least I knew I was on the right path.

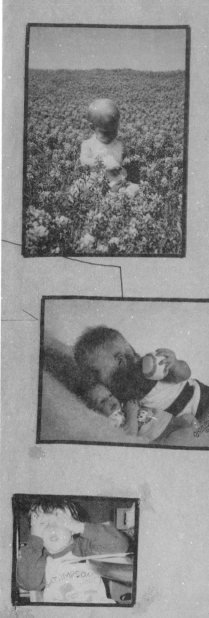

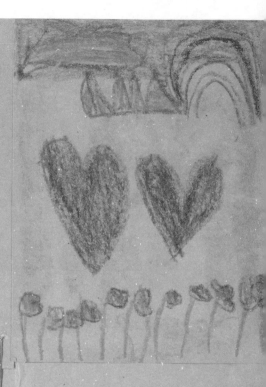

I hope you feel better real soon.

Have a good day!

Have a good sleep tonight, I hope you have good dreams.

Get well real, real, real soon.        Love,

KaLe

**"PLEASE FIGHT FOR US...
WE CANNOT FIGHT FOR OURSELVES"**

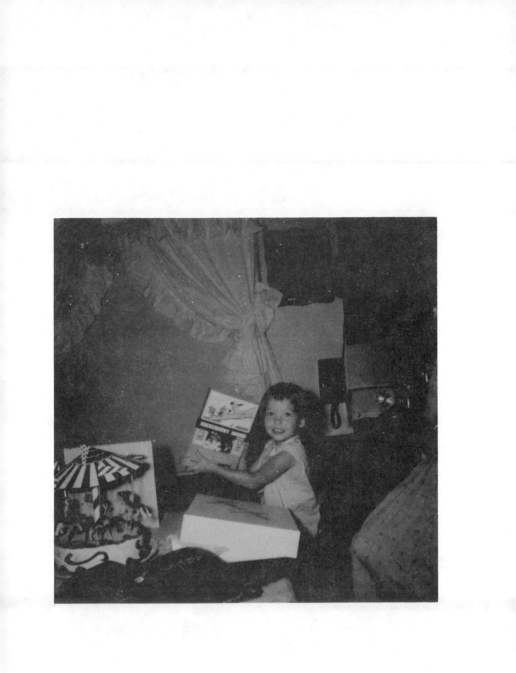

My family hopes you get well soon.

Love,

Willy

**"PLEASE FIGHT FOR US. . .
WE CANNOT FIGHT FOR OURSELVES"**

# CHAPTER FOUR

## Falling to My knees

I don't know how I was able to get up the next morning and go to work. I was emotionally drained. My eyes were puffy and swollen from crying the night before.

It was early in the day when our Executive Director called me into his office. I thought, "Oh, my God. I'm going to be fired." In my position it was imperative that I was "up" most of the time. When you teach motivation, it helps to be motivated yourself. If I had not had years of practice at "faking it" I probably would have been fired a few months earlier.

I tried to find out from his secretary what he wanted, but she didn't know. She didn't think it was anything to be alarmed about. "Christine, why are you so worried?" she asked.

Why was I so worried? After my experience the night before, I felt that everyone could see through me. I had no idea who I was. I was that frightened little girl I had always been. Since I now recognized that fact, I was sure that everyone else would see through me too.

Every day I would see the Executive Director. I discussed work plans with him. It shouldn't be any different now. I walked into his office and did the only thing that I knew how to do. I put that smile on my face and said, "Good Morning, Mr. Andrews. How are you?" I was back to my "normal self." We visited for a few minutes and then I returned to my office.

He had called me into his office to ask me to teach a stress management seminar for the administrative staff at the local community college. I said, "Oh, sure, I'd love to. Thank you so much for asking me!"

I wanted to laugh. He was asking me to teach a stress management course. Here was this person that was about to have a nervous breakdown, if she had not already had one. I had fever blisters and ulcers in my mouth, and had bruises all over my body which probably meant that my leukemia was coming back. And he called me a stress management "expert."

I taught the course that week. The strangest thing happened. I put on my "Ms. Motivation" face, got the audience fired up and involved, but I was also myself. I told them the truth. I confessed to them about my experience and the pain that I was going through with Joe. I told them about the mouth ulcers. I discovered that I didn't have to be perfect to teach a course. I didn't even have to necessarily have it working in my life. I just had to know the principles, deliver them in an effective manner and try to follow them myself. Their own lives would be the test of truth. They didn't have to look at my life for the answers.

Two new counselors had started working for me the week after Joe moved out. One of them was a tremendous help in my life. She was a graduate student working on her degree in Counseling. Although she had little experience, she had a very natural gift in the area of counseling. We became very close. Kelly knew what it was like to hide behind other people's problems. She had experienced the same dysfunction with her own life. We met everyday so I could guide her in handling the cases of the employees whom she was counseling. After our meeting, I then met with her for an additional hour myself. During our sessions, she assigned homework for me to do and I made commitments to myself concerning Joe.

For the first time since Joe left, I was working on my problems. I was focusing on me. I made a decision not to drive by Joe's apartment anymore. I didn't feel a need for Al-A-non since it dealt with the family of the alcoholic. The addict that I was concerned with now was myself. I had released Joe. I knew I was an addict when I went through withdrawals while trying to break behavior patterns. It was the most difficult thing I had ever done. Giving up something in life is tremendously different than letting it go. Letting something go requires an act of your will when you have absolutely no desire to have it gone in the first place.

I thought about the analogy of a bird in a cage. If the bird somehow got loose and flew away and never came back. . . I would have no choice but to give it up. Letting the bird go would require much more action on my part. Knowing that the bird would be better off where it could flap it's wings and reach it's full potential, even if it meant that it may be hurt or possibly die. . . letting go would be opening the door and sending it to find it's own destiny.

The twelve steps were becoming more important to me each day. Even though I was no longer attending Al-A-non, I still tried to work a 12-step program. I attended a CODA (Co-Dependents Anonymous) meeting, but I was not ready for that group. Everyone was talking about themselves so freely. They didn't have any one else attached to their addiction like Al-A-non. I did great at opening up as long as I could drag someone or something in with me. I could go to Alcoholics Anonymous and talk about my tendency toward alcoholism. I was comfortable in Sex and Love Addicts Anonymous where I could talk about Joe being my addiction, but I wasn't ready to show the world that I did not have a self. I didn't know what role to play when I went to that group. So, I didn't go. I later learned that is what my addiction is all about. . . playing a role.

It had been a week since I had "broken my vows." When I awoke in the morning, my bruises were gone. I ran my tongue along the inside of my lip. There were no fever blisters in my mouth.

I didn't understand where I was going, but I knew I was on the right path. More than anything, I wanted to <u>live.</u> Once again I was climbing uphill. I wanted so desperately to reach the mountain top. I thought, "If I can just stay on the path. . . one step at a time."

I was learning many things about myself. It seemed that everyday presented a different challenge. My supervisor called me into his office to tell me that our company would probably be having another major lay-off. It wasn't definite, but he wanted to let me know so I could start securing some other business contracts. I remember thinking, "Can't I just get on even ground before I get knocked off?" I had always pictured myself as a mountain climber. I never really knew what was on top, but whatever it was...I wanted it.

As the days went by, I still had not heard from Joe. I was becoming extremely vulnerable. Everyone advised me not to drive by his apartment anymore. My friends were concerned that something harmful was going to happen to me. I couldn't understand why everyone was so frightened of Joe. "There's no reason to be afraid," I said. "Joe would never hurt me. I really believe in some strange way he left because he loved me; not because he didn't love me."

A few weeks went by before I realized that although releasing myself was imperative, I still could not seek out a divorce. I didn't believe in divorce. I wanted Joe to take responsibility for filing. As much as I wanted my marriage, I wanted to go on with life, but not enough to compromise my values.

Not knowing how Joe felt was keeping me from taking action for divorce proceedings also. I had not talked to him in three months. The last thing he had said to me was, "I don't want a divorce. I'll call you on Friday." Everyday I wondered if he was going to be dead or alive. I decided I had to put some closure on the relationship. Before I did, though, I would have to hear from Joe directly that he had made his decision.

I decided to write Joe a letter.

It took me five hours to write the letter. It was dated October 31, 1989. The letter was difficult to write, but I was completely honest with him. I expressed my feelings, my fears, my own addictions and the struggle I had faced since he moved out. I confronted him about his disease. I closed the letter by saying:

> *"I love you, Baby. And God loves you.*
> *He has an incredible plan for your life. I think you know in your heart that "it's" not working for you anymore. Joe, I can't stop you from dying. All I can do is offer a hand. You may divorce me after reading this letter and that is your choice. I can't stop you from doing that anymore than I an stop you from dying. But the one thing you can NOT do is get me to stop loving you. No matter what you are involved in, you will never get me to stop loving you. You will have to go to your grave knowing that there was nothing you could do to get me to stop loving you.*
> *That's all I can do. The rest is yours. If you need me, you know where I am.*

I finished the letter. It was five pages long. There were no secrets left. I re-read it twelve times before I went to bed. I would make a copy of it the next day and put it in the mail. I was determined to get to the top of that mountain. With or without Joe, I was going to the top. I thought, "I may be dead when I get there, but I was determined that I was **going** to get there."

I arrived at work early the following morning so I could make a copy of the letter to Joe. Tim, the mail clerk, always bought stamps and mailed my personal mail for me when he stopped at the post office. I wanted to catch him before he left. I handed the envelope to him. He looked into my eyes when he saw who it was addressed to. "I'm praying for you, Christine. You just hang in there. God's going to see you through," he said. Tim worked for Joe at one time. He had changed jobs after Joe got fired.

I remembered when Joe and I were dating. Tim was so excited. He use to come into my office and tell me how much he liked Joe. Tim would talk about what Joe had done for him. Joe had apparently given him a promotion when no one else would. As those memories surfaced, I commented to him how much Joe had always thought of him. I did not want to knock Joe off of Tim's pedestal, but I knew that he would know the truth. He had talked to me about Joe when Joe first moved out.

"Tim, I need to ask you something. You don't have to answer me if you don't want to. It's okay. But was Joe using cocaine when he was working here?" I asked. I don't know how many people would have to tell me before I believed it.

"Well, I can't say for sure," Tim said. "But you know most of the guys over there "do coke" and there were rumors. And you know. . . he always went around sniffling. You know when people do that. . .I mean, no body has a runny nose year round," he continued.

I never thought about that. Joe lived with a runny nose. I found boxes of Benadril hidden under a cloth in his bathroom drawer. When I inquired as to why the boxes weren't in the medicine cabinet upstairs, where we kept our medications, he became defensive with me. It was the same day that I almost lost my hand. Joe was doing some work at the breakfast table. I was in my office working. I went to ask him a question about some plans we had made. When I reached for the calendar in his brief case, he slammed the top down. I looked at him as if he had lost his mind.

I said, "Joe. . . I just wanted to look at the calendar." He was trying to lock his briefcase.

"What do you have in there?" I asked as I started laughing. I tried to reach for the briefcase. In playful jest, Joe wrestled me to the floor. But he would not let me look inside of his briefcase. He locked it and would not open it again. And he always kept it in his car when it wasn't with him.

It was difficult to believe the man I married. . . the man that was going to be the father of my child was a cocaine user. I was a closet smoker when Joe and I became engaged. That was part of my secret world. It was not acceptable behavior in my circle of friends so I couldn't let anyone know. I wondered if that is how Joe felt. Somehow when you hide your addiction and nobody sees it, it doesn't really exist. At least you don't have to face it.

In working with Kelly, I made some decisions to put my life in order. When Joe left, it was too painful to wear my wedding ring. Since it was 2.25 carats, I did not want to leave it in my house. My dad put it in his safety deposit box at his bank. I remember when Joe put the ring on my finger. He turned it three times as if he was tightening it. He looked at me and said, "And that's where it will stay for the rest of our lives." It was the ring I always wanted, but more than that - it represented I had finally found the man that I had always wanted.

One of the decisions I made was to get my ring out of the safety deposit box. I wanted to have it reset. The ring was appraised at over $10,000.00. I knew that I could not get that price for it if I sold it. I decided to have it set as a dinner ring. I gave a deposit to the jewelerer to hold the ring. If Joe got into treatment and our marriage got back together, then I could have it put back in the original setting.

I called Dad and asked him to get my diamond out of his safety deposit box. He met me at a restaurant that night. As I looked at the ring, it looked different to me. I told Dad, "It's been a long time since I've seen this ring. I must be healing. It doesn't even look like the same ring."

I thanked Dad for dinner and drove to the jewelry store. As I handed the ring to the jeweler, all of the sales clerks gathered around and commented what a beautiful stone it was. They were very polite. Each of them asked if they could look at it.

"I don't think I have ever seen such a perfect stone," the jeweler said. "He must have paid a pretty penny for this." It never dawned on me until the jeweler made that comment where the money had come from. Joe had been out of work and had declared bankruptcy, yet he had money to buy the ring that I wanted.

I thought about the time I originally had the ring appraised. The appraiser commented on the stone. He commented on the clarity of the ring and said that it was worth $10,000. You could definitely sell it for $8500.00," he said.

I got tears in my eyes as I thought about Joe buying that ring for me. Now I would give anything to have Joe sober and have a cigar ring instead. I didn't need a diamond that size. Joe must have gotten the money from selling drugs. I was wearing a 2.25 carat diamond and Joe was dying because of it.

The jeweler was speaking to me while I was thinking about Joe. I heard the last few words of his sentence.

"I'm sorry," I said. "What did you say?"

"Do you have the appraisal with you?" he asked.

"Well, no. I didn't know I needed it. It was appraised somewhere around $10,000.00. Do I need to get the papers?" I asked.

"No, it's not necessary. However, we do have to have a value placed on the ring before we can work on it. Would you mind if I appraised it?" he asked.

"Oh, of course not. That's fine," I said.

The sales clerk and I were visiting while the jeweler appraised the stone. He was taking such a long time. I thought "Don't tell me. The ring is stolen. There is some way to trace it. Joe bought a stolen diamond." I smiled at the jeweler as he looked at me from the back room. He walked out and handed the ring to the sales clerk. He whispered something to her. They both looked at me. My heart was beating rapidly. I knew something was wrong. She mumbled something to me that I could not understand.

"I beg your pardon," I said.

"You knew that though. Didn't you?" she asked. I leaned forward to be sure that I could hear her.

"I knew what?" I asked her to repeat herself as I struggled to hear what these people were saying to me. I couldn't understand why they were talking so quietly.

Our faces were inches apart as we both leaned over the glass counter.

"It's a CZ," she said.

"It's a what?" I asked. I felt like I had gone deaf.

"It's a cubic zirconia. This stone is not a diamond." she said.

At that moment my entire body shut down. I just stared at the sales clerk. I tried to swallow but I couldn't even do that. My eyes were fixed on the mouth that had just uttered those words. After what seemed like several minutes, I pulled myself off the glass counter. I glanced down at the beautiful diamonds in the case. For the first time in my life I knew what it meant to have frozen tears. I turned around and walked out of the store.

I have no idea how I got home that night. Looking back on the experience, I must have been in total shock. I do not remember walking out of the mall. I do not remember getting in my car or driving home. It reminds me of some of my experiences in college. I would "go out partying" and have too much to drink. I would black out.

It was that way the night I found out about my ring. I don't remember anything about the night. The only thing I remember is walking to the mailbox to get my mail. For over three months I rushed home from work hoping to find a letter from Joe. Each day I would pray, "God, please let today be the day. Let there be a letter from Joe in the mailbox."

For the first time since Joe moved out hearing from him was the furthest thing from my mind. All I could think about were those words that I had heard just a short time before I arrived home... "You did know that, didn't you? It's a cubic zirconia."

I glanced through my mail. My legs became limp as I saw an envelope that was addressed with my maiden name. It was in Joe's handwriting. I walked into my office to sit down. I sat in the chair next to Joe's picture. I was opening the envelope when the phone rang. My answering machine was on. I decided I would let whoever was calling leave a message since I was not in any condition to talk to anyone. The voice on the machine was a familiar voice. I instantly knew who it was.

"Mrs. Michael, this is Pat from the jewelry store. We need to know what to do with this ring. You've given us $800.00 and we don't know what to do with it. Do you still want us to set this stone? Also, I was talking with our appraiser and he thinks that you might want to contact your attorney. If you have had your diamond cleaned or worked on, it could be the person who worked on it traded it out for the stone that you now have. He said that happens a lot. I am sorry. Please give us a call and let us know what to do," she said.

I tried desperately to fit the pieces together to determine what happened to my diamond. I thought "Could someone have gotten it out of the safety deposit box?" I was notorious for having my jewelry professionally cleaned every time I went to the shopping mall. I would drop by any jewelry store and have my jewelry cleaned. I never left it anywhere though. I would always stand by the counter and wait for it to be cleaned. A million possibilities were going through my mind as I removed the letter from the envelope.

I was right. The letter was from Joe. I looked at the envelope to see when it was mailed. The letter had been mailed two days earlier, but it was postmarked from Louisiana. The letter was written on yellow ledger paper that Joe carried in his briefcase. I tried to take a deep breath before I started reading the letter. A tear ran down my face as I began. The letter said:

*Christine,*

*I'm going to try and put down on paper my feelings and reaction to you and to your letter.*

*First, I want to let you know that I never wanted to hurt you. You are the most sensitive, caring person in the whole world and you deserve a lot better in your life than to be hooked up with me.*

*When I told Debra that you should go on with your life because it would only hurt you because of a reevaluation of my own life, I meant that I wanted to start taking control of my own life and the events in it instead of them controlling me. That's what was happening to me. It would be easy just to stay in our relationship, but it would-n't be fair to you, because I felt dead and it would eventually bring you down.*

*I had realized that I could never be what you wanted or give you what you wanted most - children. The more that I tried to adapt to your wants, the more I knew I was deceiving myself and even worse - deceiving you.*

*My love for you was very real, Christine. I have never loved anyone or anything as deeply as I loved you, but it was fading. I had become numb. I couldn't ask anymore from a woman than what you gave me. I just couldn't continue taking advantage of your love when I couldn't give you what you needed and wanted most out of life. That is why I left you.*

*I want nothing more than the best for you be-cause you deserve it. You need a man who can love you back the way that you love him, who can and wants to give you children, who can give you the home life you deserve. You can still find it, Christine. It's not me, however.*

*I'm troubled by your letter which was followed by a letter from Debra. First of all, I don't know where this "knowledge" that I am using and selling drugs came from. I don't do drugs and definitely wouldn't sell the poison. For you to even think that I would indicates that you really didn't know me.*

*The thing that I guess just reinforces my opinion about women in general is the fact that they just can't keep confidences. What I told you about me, when I bore my soul as to what and who I was, was for you only. It is hard for me to open up anyway because I am a private person. I trusted you with my feelings and told you things about my experiences that I have never told anyone. Now, I find you evidently told Debra*

*Christine, I guess the bottom line is we both need to go our separate ways. I could never forget you. You are the most wonderful and loving and caring woman in this world. I am sorry that you ever met me because I only hurt you in this relationship and you didn't deserve it.*

*If I hadn't of shown up, you would have been lot better off and would probably be with a man you could live happily ever after with. I want you to know that I have been touched by you in a way that I have never been touched before and know that I will never be touched again. I will never forget you. I wish it could work, but I know that it can't so I'm releasing you so you can become whole again.  Joe*

I slouched back in my chair and then collapsed on the floor. I had never experienced emotional pain to the depths that I was feeling it then. I literally thought I was going to die from the agony in my soul. Wherever it is in the human psyche that a person literally reaches their limit and can not handle any more grief, I knew that I was there.

I pulled myself up and gasped for air. As I sat up, I saw Joe's picture sitting on the end table. I grabbed it and through it across the room. "You liar," I screamed. "You damn liar! I loved you, Joe. You're a damn liar" I cried as I fell back to the floor. I must have sobbed for hours. All I could vocalize was "I loved you, Joe. Why? Why did you do this? Why Joe?" Those were the last words that I remember saying before I fell asleep.

It was three o'clock in the morning when I woke up. I sat straight up and looked at the clock. I was still on the floor of my office. I stared at Joe's picture lying in the corner broken into a thousand pieces. My body was paralyzed as I remembered the day that my house-keeper had found the C.D. deposit in the very room in which I was sitting. It was a deposit for $8000.00 dated on May 1, 1989. That was the same day that I went to the hospital to have my bone marrow harvested; the day that Joe "had" to be in Louisiana for a meeting. I thought about how Joe had so "protectively" asked the nurse, "Doesn't she need to take off her rings before she goes to surgery?" He couldn't stay until I went to surgery. He said he had to catch a plane that morning at 8:00 A.M. He made the deposit that morning in the suburb where we lived. Joe had sold my diamond. All the pieces fit together. "You damn liar," I thought to myself. "You're a damn liar, Joe." I knew asking "why" was futile.

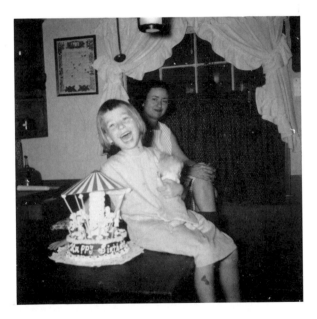

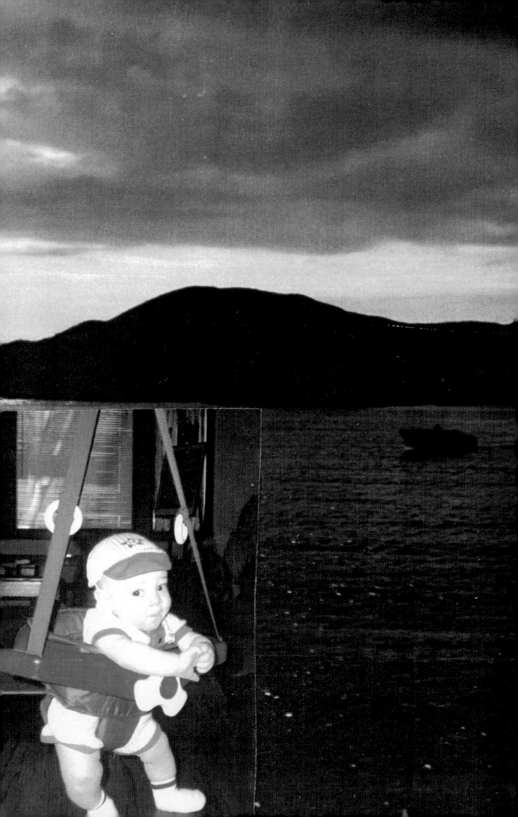

# CHAPTER FIVE

## *The Battle of Survival*

I called my supervisor that morning and told him that I would not be in to work. I must have read Joe's letter fifty times trying to find some way to put closure on my heart. Each time I read the words that were meant to release me from the relationship, I became more hooked into Joe's disease. I kept thinking, "If I could just find something to hold on to. . . if I just knew why." I repeatedly read the statement that Joe made concerning the reason he left. He realized he could never be what I wanted or give me what I wanted the most. . . a child.

Each time I read that sentence, I grabbed my stomach and thought about the baby I had lost. Joe and I were going to try to conceive again in December. That would have been the following month.

Often when I would blame myself for the failure of my marriage or when I would try to understand why Joe was not taking action for ending the marriage, I would talk to Kelly. She would say, "Christine, you're dealing with someone who is using mind altering drugs. You are trying to gain understanding from someone who doesn't have any understanding. He's mind-altered. Joe's not in control of his life. The cocaine is."

I thought about that comment and decided to call Kelly. She came over and I handed her the letter. As she finished reading it, she put her hand to her mouth. A tear rolled down her cheek.

"That's really sad," she said as tears began to flow from her eyes. "How does that make you feel?"

I echoed her comment in response. "How does that make you feel?"

"Like I was wrong," she said.

"You mean, he's not using cocaine. He just didn't love me?" The thought of that was more than I could handle. As long as I could justify Joe's actions through his disease or find some reason for his behavior, I wouldn't have to admit what I believed all along. I was unlovable.

Kelly said, "No, it's obvious that he does love you. He loves you as much as he is capable of loving anyone. He told you that in the letter. I mean, Christine, he's in denial. You uncovered his secret. It's the only thing he could do. He's running. I just thought he was a lot closer than he is. Christine, he's got a long way to go before he 'bottoms out'. He may never hit bottom until it's too late. He's got a long history of running. I am so sorry."

Both of us cried as if we were experiencing the same loss. It was always helpful to talk to Kelly. I think I would have lambasted her if she got so personally involved with any of her clients. But Kelly and I had become good friends. Not only was she an excellent counselor, but she had used cocaine in the past and knew drug dealers in our city. She could often put the pieces together for me.

Although I knew the truth on a cognitive level, emotionally I felt I was still to blame. I felt rejected and felt that somehow I deserved what happened to me. It didn't matter who told me differently. I heard from several sources what I should believe to be fact. My reality, however, was ingrained in the depth of my being. . . I was unlovable.

I spent the remainder of the day packing Joe's things. I took the cards he had given me, the letters he had written and all the pictures I had of him and put them in a box. I placed everything in the downstairs closet and closed the door to that part of my life.

My mind was tormented by a comment that Joe made in his letter. He had written, "For you to think that I would [use and sell drugs], indicates you really didn't know me." The other comment that bothered me was, "The thing that reinforces my opinion about women in general is the fact that they just can't keep confidences." The more I thought about that suggestion, the more irate I became. I had not told Debra anything that Joe had not told her himself.

Joe could leave me, but he was not going to leave me without hearing the truth. I went to my office and typed a three page letter to him. I closed the letter by saying, "One day you are going to look in the mirror and see the people that hurt you the most. You are going to see that you have turned out exactly like your mother and father. Because you refuse to let them go. You have buried them inside of you. They're not dead, Joe. They're living inside of you and living through your life. Joe, you are the only one that can do anything about it. I think that you know in your heart, Baby, how very much that I love you. I have not written these things to hurt you. I have written these things because I want so much for the pain to be over. I will let you go. It is your decision. I just could not end this relationship knowing that I didn't fight for the most important thing in my life; not my marriage, but YOU. I will give up on my marriage, but I will never give up on you. You will have to leave the face of the Earth before I ever quit praying for you and believing that somehow, someday Joey will return to himself and have the life that God so desperately wants to give him. I will always love you, Joe. You are now free."

The date of that letter was November 20, 1989. I put the letter in an envelope, addressed it and drove to the post office. I stood by the mailbox for several minutes. I looked at the envelope. I knew as soon as I let go of that letter there was no getting it back. I also knew that it would be the last time that Joe and I had any communication. Joe was gone forever. I prayed every day on the way to work that I would be served with divorce papers. I found myself rushing home at night so that I could be there when the deputy sheriff arrived.

I could not understand why Joe would not take action to end the marriage. Why would someone that wanted out of a relationship not get out? If he no longer loved me, why wouldn't he file for divorce? I had told him in my letter that I didn't want anything from him and that I would pay for all court costs and attorney fees. Each day I awaited the arrival of divorce papers. They never came.

Within two weeks from the time I received Joe's letter, I was showing signs of relapsing with leukemia. The following month I was passing clots the size of racquetballs. My gums were bleeding profusely and I had six-inch-by-ten-inch bruises all over my body.

The night I released myself from my marriage by going through the motions of breaking my vows almost killed me. Now I knew no matter how much I wanted Joe to file for divorce - no matter how much I wanted him to take responsibility for his decision, I could not hold on any longer. I was literally going to die.

It was time for my normal three month check up with my oncologist. The blood tests reinforced my biggest fear and proved what I had already known. My blood counts were abnormal. The doctor left me in the examination room while he went to view my blood sample in the lab. When he returned he had a relieved look on his face. He said, "Well, I feel a little better. I didn't see any cancer cells in the peripheral blood, but I still want to do a biopsy as soon as possible." He scheduled the biopsy for the following day.

Immediately upon returning to my office, I called my attorney. I made an appointment for 12:00 noon, two hours before my biopsy. During our meeting I commented to him, "There is no way that we will catch Joe at home. How can we serve him papers?" He inquired about his schedule.

"Larry," I said, "Joe is never home. When he's working, he travels. I want out of this marriage the fastest, easiest, most painless way possible. I don't want anything from him. I'll pay for everything. I just want to live," I said as I began to cry.

My attorney told me that he could send Joe a waiver of citation, but unlike divorce papers it had to be signed. "I can send it through the mail by certified mail, but according to law he has to sign it, Christine. Do you think that Joe will sign the waiver?"

I said, "At this point, I think Joe would do anything for me." The law required that I wait 60 days before going to court. I couldn't stand the thought of waiting any longer while a deputy sheriff chased Joe down. It could take weeks to find him.

"Send the waiver," I said. The original petition for divorce was filed on December 4, 1989 at 3:29 P.M. My attorney told me he would call me when he received the signed paper. The only request I had was that he did not appear in court due to my health.

I went immediately from the meeting with my attorney to the scheduled appointment with my doctor. I never allowed my doctor to do the biopsy unless we told jokes the entire time. This time it was difficult to even muster a smile.

My dear friend, Debra, had agreed to meet me at the doctor's office. She held my hand during the biopsy, but Dr. Douglas was his usual self. He always made me laugh and had a unique way of making things better; no matter how bleak they were in reality. He had been my strength in fighting the battle of cancer when I was first diagnosed. Now, when my entire life was in shambles, he still would not let me forget. . . laughter is the best medicine.

I received a phone call from Dr. Douglas the following day. He had gotten the biopsy results back. The test were inconclusive. He wanted to do another biopsy. It was late in the day so I did not go back to work. Over dinner with a friend, I explained to her the results of the biopsy.

"Christine, your mouth. . . " she said in a whisper. She covered her eyes in disgust. I reached up and touched my mouth with a napkin. It was pouring with blood. I put my head down and covered my face with my hands. I tried to hide the tears when I heard my friend say, "Christine, I'm sorry, but I just can't handle this. I can not go through this again with you." As I looked up, she was reaching for the check. "You know, sometimes it's just really hard to be your friend. I can't handle the thought of losing you," she said. I sat in disbelief as I watched her wipe her eyes, slide out of the booth and leave the restaurant. I tried to call her from a pay phone at the restaurant. I tried again when I arrived home. She would not answer the phone and would not return my calls. She never did.

I went upstairs and laid on my bed for hours. I thought about my life and wondered why I fought so hard to live. As I got ready for bed, I stood in front of the mirror and gasped when I saw the new bruises that had developed that day. I turned around and looked at the reflection of the back of my legs. I sighed heavily and said, "Hang on, Christine."

I threw on a pair of "sweats", got in my car and drove to the store. I bought three pairs of dark colored panty hose to cover the bruises on my legs. As I stood in line, I thought about my friend running out of the restaurant. That was the fourth time that one of my closest friends had ended our relationship during my battle with cancer. It was as if they thought that the disease was contagious. I thought to myself, "Every single person that was at my "wedding" is gone. My closest friends had stood by me when I was so hurt by my family. Now they were gone too.

I smiled at the cashier at the check-out stand.

"How are you?" she asked.

"I'm doing great," I said. "Thanks for asking. How are you?"

"I'm a little tired," she replied.

"Yeah, me too," I said as I reached out and touched her arm. "Have a good evening. Okay?"

I looked into the night sky as I walked to my car.

"God," I said, "I don't care if I lose every friend that I have. Joe can walk out on me and this life can take everything away from me. But it's not going to have me! God, you told me you were adding fifteen years to my life. It hasn't even been eighteen months. Oh **God, I want to live!!!**" I cried out from the bottom of my heart. I then began to laugh. "I don't exactly know why, Lord, but I want to live."

As I started to slide back into illness, I saw myself as a child again. At age 3, I began to have severe bladder and kidney problems. Two years later, I was hospitalized for sixteen days while my urologist reconstructed my bladder. My mother never left my side. I don't think she ever went home to change clothes during that entire time. Dad would bring her things to the hospital, but she wouldn't leave. I remember being wheeled off to surgery. The anesthesiologist had administered a pre-med before taking me to the operating room. I was screaming in terror.

As the medication began to take effect, I thought I saw my mother standing behind me talking with a nurse. As the attendants proceeded to wheel me through the double doors, I screamed "Mommy, don't leave me." I saw her look toward me, look back to the nurses that she was in conversation with and laugh. She just stood there and watched me as I tried to escape from the table in which I was strapped.

It was not until my adult life I discovered that event never happened. My mother went to the operating room with me. She remembers me screaming. However, she was the one crying the most and saying "Please, let me go with her." Somehow in my mind, though, I was being punished. I had not been good enough and my parents were going to give me away. It seemed the only time I was allowed to be "me" was when I was sick. The whole world stopped when I became ill. The pressures were taken off. I didn't have to be a "good little girl." I could cry when I hurt, laugh and play to my heart's content and never get in trouble for it. Memories of my childhood illnesses haunted me as I fought a constant battle to live. I was having blood tests and bone marrow biopsies approximately every two days. Each test would come back with the same results. The tests were inconclusive.

My doctor sent the lab report and slides to numerous hospitals, pathologists and oncologists around the country. They all said the same thing, "We don't understand what this could be. They look like leukemic cells, but they are not doing anything. If it was a relapse, she should have relapsed by now. The marrow only shows what appears in the blood a few days later. Let's just keep watching it."

Every time I received the report from the biopsy, I was ecstatically happy. Then, my blood counts would start to drop   Then - they would rise and return to normal.   After a few weeks of this rollercoaster type experience, I started to look to my Bible for answers. If there was an answer available, I was going to find it. I tried to make sense out of what was happening to me. I knew that it wasn't "God's will" for me to relapse and I knew that it certainly wasn't "my will," so there had to be an answer.

Every verse I opened to had something to say about a bruise. I read in the book of Isaiah, Chapter 30: "In quietness and trust is your strength. . . He will surely be gracious to you at the sound of your cry; when He hears it, He will answer you.   Although the Lord has given you bread of privation and water of oppression, He, your teacher will no longer hide Himself, but your eyes will behold your Teacher.   And your ears will hear a word behind you, "This is the way, walk in it, whenever you turn to the right or to the left."

"  . .*Whenever you turn to the right or to the left. . .*" Those words stuck in my mind. I read on. "And you will defile your graven image.   You will scatter them as an impure thing and say to them, "Be Gone!"   Then He will give you rain for the seed which you will sow in the ground, and bread from the yield of the ground and it will be rich and plenteous on that day that the Lord binds up the fracture and *heals the **bruise** that He has inflicted.*" I started to pray. "God, that blows me away," I said. Of all things for me to read about . . the thing in which I am most afraid.   You say in your Word that you will heal the bruise.   Are you saying that you are going to heal me?" I asked.

I began to meditate and pray. I heard a voice within me say, "Christine, do not look to the left and do not look to the right. Just look straight into my eyes." For some reason, I turned to the Book of Jeremiah and went directly to Chapter 30. . ."For thus says the Lord, Your bruise is incurable, and your injury is serious. . . No healing for your sores. Your lovers have forgotten you. . . " I began to laugh. "This is ridiculous," I thought until I glanced down at a verse that I had underlined. It was verse 17 which stated, "For I will restore you to health And I will heal you of your bruises, declares the Lord."

I said to God: "I don't have that kind of faith. I've faked it all my life. Everyone thinks that I am such a 'woman of God', but I'm not. I'm just me, God and I am so tired. I love you, but I am so scared. I don't want to die."

". . . Do not look to the left or to the right, but look into my eyes." That quote ran over and over in my mind. I looked in the concordance of the Bible to see if there were any other verses that said the same thing. There was one in Deuteronomy. It said "and do not turn aside from any of the words which I commanded you today, to the right or to the left, to go after other gods to serve them. If you do...You will be stricken on your legs with sore boils that cannot be healed because you would not obey the Lord your God by keeping His command- ment." I was reading to get comfort and instead I was getting threatened by God. Didn't He understand how difficult it was for me to believe? I decided to call a church that had prayed for me before. Maybe they could get through to Him. I wasn't having much luck. I told the woman who answered the phone what was happening in my life.

She prayed with me and then said "Christine, there is a verse I want you to read. It is Jeremiah 30:17. It says 'For I will restore you to health and I will heal your bruises, declares the Lord'. He's healing you. You just have to trust Him." Christine, you are not to look to the left or to the right. He means what He says when He tells you He is going to restore you to health. Don't get in His way. He doesn't need your help." I could not believe what I was hearing. I had never met this woman. She did not know me. She didn't know I had just spent the last two hours in prayer and reading my Bible. The verse she gave me was the same verse I had read before I called her. I was dumbstruck. I shared with her about the experience I had just minutes before I called her. "I called you," I said, "because I thought maybe you could get through to Him better than I could." She laughed as if she was somewhat surprised herself.

"That's the Lord," she said. "He means what He says." As I hung up the phone, I sat in amazement of what had just happened. I thought to myself, "God, you really do meet us exactly where we are."

At that moment I heard His voice say, "Christine, I wouldn't blame you if you never trusted me again. But, I promise, if you just hang with Me and just trust Me, I promise I am going to give back to you seven times seventy what has been taken from you." He didn't say ten-fold as I had always been taught, but seven times seventy. It was the same number as the Bible commands us to forgive others. . . seven times seventy.

I always thought I had to be perfect to have God love me. Now He was saying that all He wanted was my trust. When it came to prayer, my philosophy was "If the prayers of one righteous man availeth much, the prayers of 5000 does a whole lot more." I called every church with a "prayer ministry" that was listed in the yellow pages. I called my friend in Houston and asked him to do the same thing. My friend in El Paso promised to do her part. We had Texas covered. Any time someone would call from another state I asked them to have their church pray. Many churches had people scheduled around the clock to pray. Every time that someone asked if they could pray with me on the phone inevitably they would close by saying the same thing. . . "do not look to the left or to the right. Just keep your eyes on Jesus"

But the Bible wasn't the only place I searched for answers. When I was in recovery I picked up a monthly magazine that listed seminars on "twelve-step programs". Whenever there was a seminar pertaining to healing I would attend. I continued visualization exercises.  My days were filled with listening to subliminal tapes on healing. The music was peaceful and of "new age" quality. I even started a macrobiotic diet.

When I arrived home for the day, I decided to do some fervent praying.  I laid down on the floor with my face buried in the carpet. I was in a prone position with my arms above my head.  I pleaded with God to hear my prayer. "God, search my heart, Lord Jesus! If there is **anything** I am holding on to that is preventing me from being healed, reveal that to me, God.  Lord, your Word says that if we confess our sins one before another then we will be healed.  If there is anyone that I have hard feelings toward or am harboring unforgiveness in my heart, reveal that to me, God. I want to live."
To my amazement. . . approximately 30 faces appeared in my mind. I pulled myself up and ran to my desk.  I got a piece of paper and a pen and began to write down the names of each person that came to mind.  The remainder of the evening was spent writing letters to each individual that I had hurt in some way. As I was writing, I remember thinking, "You know, I never did anything to these people.  They are actually the ones who hurt me. . . I was the victim," but I continued to write.  As I look back on that event I find it quite humorous.  I know half the people who received those letters thought, "What the heck is she talking about?"  The other half were probably asking themselves, "Who is Christine Michael?" Although I am somewhat "humbled" by my confession, Joe also received a letter from me.  I asked him for *his* forgiveness.

Each day became increasingly difficult. I began to hate the pat answers that everyone gave me. "Just give it to Jesus," I would hear repeatedly. "You have to stand against the enemy, Christine." I wanted to say, "Why do I have to stand against the enemy? Why can't God do it?" I was so tired of having to perform. Nothing good could happen in my life unless I said the right thing or did the right thing. I had been to counselors, healing seminars, I did guided imagery and relaxation exercises faithfully. I was on the prayer list of at least fifty churches. I had eaten whole foods until I was about to regurgitate. I had been prayed over, stood over and leaned over. I had holy oil placed on my forehead and I had been slain in the spirit.

I had people telling me that I had a curse that had been placed on my life from the third generation back. That was easy enough for me to believe. So what did I do? I went to a deliverance minister. I paid the man $50.00 to have demonic spirits cast out of my life. People were telling me that I had gotten out from God's protective umbrella and I needed to join their church to be restored. One person told me that I was living in sin by getting a divorce - I needed to reconcile with my husband so God could heal me.

One night, I finally had all I could stand. I went home, put my long satin robe on and sat on my staircase. I often sat at the top of my staircase when I reached "the end of my rope". I loved my house. When I sat at the top of my stairs, I could see most of the lower story of my home. It was very open and built with cathedral ceilings. My house was so peaceful. My house was full of country primitive antiques, with red and blue accents. My house had so much of the real me in it. I loved to just sit on my staircase and think.

As I sat on the step, I said, "God, I don't know what else to do. I have been stuck and probed so many times. I am sick of it. I have had things laid on me, taken out of me, wrapped around me and lifted off of me. I have been told to stand up, sit down, turn around . . God, I just want to live, damn it, **I want to live!!**"

I heard a voice within me speak. It was intelligible and made sense to me. The voice said, "Then quit killing yourself, Christine. Just rest." I contemplated that thought. It was then that I realized, although it made a lot of sense, I didn't know how to rest. I looked at the bruises on my arms and legs and thought to myself, "Yeah, just rest." I had lost my husband, I had lost my baby, I had almost lost my life so many times that I could no longer count them. I was told I would probably not have a job any longer. If I relapsed, I would have to have a bone marrow transplant. And then I'd be sterile for life. . .

I said, "God, you know, I would do that. . . but I have absolutely no idea what you are talking about. I feel like I am in the ring with Mike Tyson. It's the heavy weight championship and I'm Pee-Wee Herman. Everytime I get up and try to have faith, I keep getting knocked down to the ground." As I thought about that allegory, I heard the same voice within me say, "You know, if you were smart, you'd stay down for the count." I laughed when I heard that statement.

"Well, Christine, it's happened. You have totally lost it." I thought to myself. "You are either hearing voices or God has turned in to a jokester."

"If you stay down - he can't get you, Christine. You see that as giving up. To you. . . that is failure. It means that you don't have enough faith to believe that I can heal you. I never asked you to fight your own battles. I love you, Christine. You must choose to believe. You are the master of your own destiny, you determine the delineation of your faith. It has been that way from the beginning."

I couldn't comprehend at that point in my life that the God who had spoken to me the night that I was diagnosed with leukemia was the same God who spoke to me that night. When He said, "Christine, I will never leave you, nor forsake you," he meant it. From that day on, everytime I became frightened or saw another bruise, I would say to myself, "Sorry, I'm not fighting this round. You can take that up with my God. You may have defeated me, Satan. You have knocked the stuffing out of me and taken away everything in life that is precious to me. But, you know what, I have a God that you will NEVER defeat."

For six weeks the doctors were baffled. They could not understand why I was showing abnormal cells in the bone marrow when the blood test showed no signs of leukemia. It was as if someone or something had its hand on my blood keeping my cancer from coming back.

I was now laying in the middle of a boxing ring deactivated from the battle of life. I was fatally wounded and had no strength to continue my walk of faith. It was as if God had His angels stationed around my body. The darts would continue to soar toward me, but each blow was devoid of any sting.

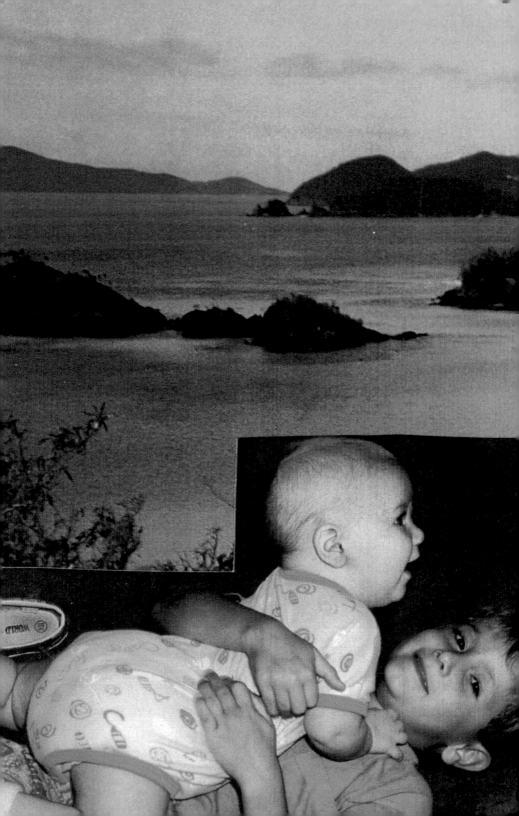

# CHAPTER SIX

## A Reason to Live

It was Christmas Eve of 1989. Attending the Christmas Eve service at my parents' church was a tradition in our family. Every year we would go and pretend to be so joyous. We would put on our smiley faces and show the world what wonderful Christians we were. Someone would always wind up in a fight and I would retrieve into my own little fantasy world.

In my fantasy world, my Christmas was always happy. It would be just like the candlelight service on Christmas Eve: Each person had a candle. They would turn to the person sitting beside them and light the wick of their candle.

As the sanctuary was lit with the "flame of love," we would sing from the bottom of our hearts. Everyone was so full of love. I wanted so much for that to be my life.

A few days before Christmas, I started hemorrhaging and passing blood clots. I was having to go to the hospital for blood tests and biopsies just about every day. I was staying at my parents' house because it was just a few blocks from the hospital.

I dressed to go to the Christmas eve service. I was wearing the same dress I had worn the previous year. It was a long red dress with full length sleeves- I wore it with my black boots so no one could see my bruises. I thought about the year before. I didn't have any bruises. I remember everyone being so excited to see Joe and me. Many people commented to Joe about how impressed they were with his faith.

"I know it hasn't been easy for you, Joe" they would say. "I bet this is the best Christmas present that you could have," as they reached out to give me a hug. Joe seemed so happy then. I couldn't hold back the tears. Christmas always meant so much to me.

When I walked into the church I could feel Joe's presence. I glanced over to where we sat the year before. I could visualize both of us sitting in the pew laughing and looking into each others' eyes. I suddenly felt like an outsider. It was as though I was invisible. I was watching everything that was going on. I could see and hear everyone around me but none of them could see me. Once again, I was standing with my nose pressed against the window of the candy store; wanting something that I would never be able to have.

Everyone was so happy that night. It was the way I always fantasized it to be. Individuals were greeting each other with hugs and kisses. The magic of Christmas was in the air. I always played the part of the "spirit of Christmas" but that year I could no longer pretend.

As the congregation began the custom of "lighting the world with just one spark," the person next to me leaned over and lit the candle that I was holding. She then reached out and touched my hand. She said, "Merry Christmas." As I turned to my mother to continue the precedence that had been set, I looked into her eyes and then looked at my dad. They both had their little respectful smiles on their faces as they played the part of having such a merry Christmas. I wanted to slap my mother as I thought about the many times that I had reached out to her for love. All I ever got from her was, "Christine, people don't like to be around people that are depressed." And my dad would just sit there. He wouldn't know a feeling if it came and sat on his head. I thought about the many times that Dad would storm out of the room at Christmas. Every year I would wind up in tears begging him to come back. But - we would always go to the Christmas eve service to "celebrate the birth of Jesus."

I looked around the room. There was NO ONE that had any idea what I was going through. Tears were flowing down my cheeks. I looked at my mother and said, "I can't do this!" I handed her my candle and ran out of the church. As I ran into the parking lot, I heard my mother's voice calling behind me.

"Christine, wait," she screamed. "Bob, go get her!" My dad was always laid back and let me go until my mother started screaming. I remember when I was in junior high I would have drastic fights with my parents. My preteen years were full of rebellion. My dad would give his typical screaming speech.

"Christine, you go to your room immediately. I will **not** put up with this disrespect. The Bible says you are to **honor** your father and mother," he would scream.

I always had the same comeback. "Yeah and it also says, "Fathers, do not provoke your children to anger." I knew the Bible too. Of course, he would remind me that the passage first commanded children to honor their parents. By the time that he was getting into his justification for yelling at me, I would scream something totally out of line and run out of the house.

I didn't really have anywhere that I wanted to go so I would sneak back into the house and hide in my closet for hours. I had a huge walk in closet that had enough things in it to keep me entertained for a lengthy period of time. I would listen as my parents would argue.

"Bob, go look for her," my mother would say. She would be in tears. "Something could happen to her. You go find her."

My dad would never do it. He would yell back at her. "I'm not going to go look for her. When she decides to come home, she will come home."

Mother would get in her car and go look for me. She would be gone for about fifteen minutes. She would come into the house calling my name. "Christine, are you home? Bob, has she come back?"

After a while I would get bored or want to go to bed. I would sneak down the stairs, open the door as if I were just coming in, shut it loud enough where I knew my parents could hear me and "storm" upstairs. By that time they were so relieved I was home they wouldn't yell at my anymore. They were just happy I was home. That is all I ever wanted from them. I didn't care about the material things they gave me. I just wanted their love.

I had left my coat in the church when I ran out. My hands were turning red from the wintry night air. My dad caught up to me to be followed by my mother. They grabbed me and pulled me next to them.

"It's okay, Sweet-heart" my mother said.

"I can't do it anymore," I said. "I can't take anymore. I am so tired of fighting." I cried as I fell to the ground. My dad caught me. "I can't do it anymore," I moaned.

Both my parents had tears in their eyes. They helped me in to the car. My mother sat in the back seat with me. She held my body that was hobble with grief. She pushed my artificial hair weave out of my face. My hair had not grown out from the first time I was sick. She stroked my face as I continued to cry.

We arrived at my parents house. I could hear the electric garage door opener pull the garage door open. My dad drove the car into the garage.

"Bob, get her out," my mother said.

"I can get myself out," I replied as I pulled away from her embrace.

"Christine, why don't you get something to eat? We have this beautiful Christmas dinner," she said.

I was so disgusted with their easy solutions. It was as if eating was the answer to the world's problems. If I ate a balanced meal, went to church and Sunday School and kept smiling - then I would always be happy. If I followed that formula, do good and be good, then God would bless me.

I knew if I relapsed with leukemia my only chance for survival would be a bone marrow transplant. I had no match in my family. That meant my chance of finding a donor was 1:20,000. Even if I did find a donor, I was having difficulty finding a reason to hold on and fight. I had an intense desire to live but I could not figure out why. I felt as though the room was spinning and I had nothing to hold on to. The one thing that I could not deal with was knowing that if I had a bone marrow transplant, I would be sterile for life. All my dreams of having a baby would be gone forever. Ironically, the reason that Joe supposedly left me was to give me the chance to have children and to have a family life that he did not want. Now I was losing that chance forever.

When I work with cancer patients I tell them that it is imperative that they view their treatment as their best friend. I could only see mine as my enemy. The procedure that was saving my life was taking away my every reason for wanting to live.

I laid on my parents bed and cried for hours. They stayed by my side. My dad was on his knees holding my hands and my mother was lying behind me with her body pressed against mine. She was holding me as tightly as she could trying to give me the security I desperately needed.

"I feel like I have been on surveillance for weeks. It's like you <u>know</u> someone is going to come and kill you," I sobbed. "You just don't know when. Every day and every night I stay awake, looking over my shoulder, just waiting. I am so tired. It would be easier if it just came back. I can't fight anymore," I cried. My parents held me miserly as if they were going to lose me if they let go.

"You don't have to fight anymore," my mother said. "We're right here. Your dad and I will fight for you. Won't we, Bob?"

"Of course we will, Sweet-heart. My dad's voice cracked as he reached out to kiss me on the forehead. "I love you," he said. He wiped his eyes as tears starting streaming down his face. I never saw my dad cry like he did that night. He had "teared up" at his brother's funeral and I saw a tear in his eye when he was told that he had cancer in 1975. I loved my dad so much. To see him hurt tore me apart.

"I don't want to die," I screamed as I buried my face in their pillow. "I don't want to die!"

My mother grabbed me and forced me to look her in the eye. "Christine, you look at me," she yelled. Her tone of voice was filled with intensity. Christine, you are *not* going to die! Do you understand me? We are going to take this one day at a time and I *promise* you one thing, little girl, I am going to be there *every* day to see you through this. And you are *not* going to die, damn it, because I'm not going to let you!" She laughed as she realized what she had said.

"I mean it," she said. "Isn't that right, Bob?"

My dad echoed her response. "That's right, Sweet-heart. You have come too far to give up now. We are going to be right there with you. You are going to make it," he told me. He then looked at me and smiled. If only things were that simple.

I realized that night there was nothing in this world that could fill the void that was so vast in my life. Nothing is lonelier than being amidst a large group of people and feeling totally isolated. I decided I would drive home and spend the evening by myself. As I drove home, I thought about all the Christmas cards I received, the parties I had been invited to and all the friends that had reached out to me in such a giving way. It was as if none of it mattered. There was an emptiness inside of me that no one could fill.

I arrived home and immediately went to the downstairs bedroom, the room that was going to be the nursery for the baby. I looked at the wallpaper filled with teddy bears and little red hearts. The top of the room had wooden shelves that would hold a collection of teddy bears. I then opened the dresser drawer and removed a picture of the crib and furniture I had bought for the baby. Joe had returned the furniture when the baby died. The crib, layette and dresser was made out of walnut. The bed was built with a canopy of white lace and had a comforter to match. It had little country blue pillows just the right size for an infant to hold. I grabbed a teddy bear from the shelf and began to cry. I thought about the day my doctor told me the baby had died. I could still feel the pain.

The thought of never being able to have another child seemed to destroy any strength I had left to undergo a marrow transplant. I had talked with adoption agencies. The verdict was always the same, "Well, with your medical history. . . I could never adopt. "Oh, Dear God, I have **nothing** to fight for!"

After hours of uncontrollable crying, I suddenly saw a little boy's face appear. He looked to be about fifteen months old; the same age that my child would have been had he lived. He had blonde hair and bright blue eyes. He looked very much like what I had imagined my baby to look like.

As I looked into this precious face, I heard a voice say, "Mommy, please don't give up. I love you. I need you to fight for me!" Immediately, other children's pictures appeared with his. They were all saying the same thing. "Please don't give up! We can't fight. Please fight for us!" they cried.

Somehow it was as if God knew the love in my heart for my baby was the only thing I had left. I had fought so hard to save his life. Now he was fighting to save mine. He would live through me and through the lives of many other children, but I had to choose to go on. I had to fight for them because they could not fight for themselves.

I thought about how upset Joe would get when I talked to other people about my experience with cancer and losing the baby. He wanted to bury it like Joe buried everything else in his life. We would always get into an argument as I would say, "Joe, we're losing over 10,000 lives a year because people can't find a donor. Many of those lives are children.", I would scream. Whenever I thought about a little child having leukemia or another potentially fatal disease it did not matter what obstacle was in my way. Each of us have a child within us. Each of us have a right to live."

I closed my eyes and tried to visualize the face of the child that appeared to me, but it was gone. All I had before were the memories that I had created in my mind. That night, however, I had seen my son. It was not something that I created in my mind. It was something that lived in my heart.

I looked at my dog and said, "Valentine, we're going to make it." I went upstairs and went to bed.

The following morning I got up to discover I was bleeding. I took a deep breath, took a shower and got dressed. As I brushed my teeth, my gums bled profusely. I was still passing blood clots. I looked at myself in the mirror and said, "Sorry, honey, it's Christmas. This can wait until tomorrow."

I spent the day by myself. I took long walks in the cool breeze. I drove to the park to feed the ducks. My parents called and wanted me to go to my aunt's house for dinner. I couldn't do it. I didn't want everyone feeling sorry for me. I wanted more than anything to be happy; just for once to have a Christmas where everyone was full of joy. I thought about Joe a lot that day. He always hated Christmas. He always wanted to pretend it didn't exist. I knew he probably would spend Christmas by himself. His kids always went to their mother's house on holidays. That afternoon I drove by Joe's apartment. I had not been there in several weeks. I turned on his street and parked by the curb. I could see his glass sliding door where I had watched him come in so many nights. He would always be by himself and go straight to the refrigerator to get a beer. And then he would go sit in the dark and watch T.V. I got tears in my eyes. "Oh, Joe," I thought, "you had *so* much. You had *so* much!"

"I'm sorry, Baby. I loved you with everything inside of me. But you've got to love yourself or it just doesn't work. Goodbye Joe" I said. I took a deep breath, but this time the air was filled with peace. I drove off and never looked back. I had a purpose. That purpose was not found in someone else. It was inside of my own heart.

The day after Christmas I woke up with a tranquility I had never experienced in my life. I could feel the sunlight on my face as it revealed the life around me. Valentine was awake and greeted me with the kisses of sunrise as he did each morning. I snuggled deep within my bed as I felt the cool air of the winter dawn. I loved to sleep with the window open just a small bit and curl up on my antique feather mattress enwrapped by my lush country comforter. I looked out the bay windows of my bedroom and heard the birds singing. There was so much life around me. More importantly, though, there was life *inside* of me.

I went to the phone and called my father.

"Dad," I said, "It's time to go to the hospital. I've relapsed."

"Christine, you don't know that for sure. If you want to go have a blood test, I'll take you to the hospital," he said. He immediately came over.

"What makes you think that you've relapsed?" he inquired.

I twisted my waist to where he could see the back of my legs. I lifted my robe. Dad got tears in his eyes as he saw what I had discovered during my shower. My entire right hip was bruised. There was not once inch of clear flesh that could be seen. My smile revealed bleeding gums and thick masses of blood over my teeth. My dad winced as he saw what the disease had done in such a short period of time.

"What do you want to do, Christine? Do you want to go to the doctor's office or do you want to go straight to the hospital?" he asked.

"You know what I really want to do? I want to go have breakfast." I said. "I want the biggest breakfast we can find. I want gravy and biscuits and all that stuff with high cholesterol that you shouldn't eat," I said. "By God, if I'm going to die. . . I'm going to have a good time doing it."

As my dad and I sat at the restaurant, we talked about life and we talked about death. It was something we had never discussed on a personal level. We had many philosophical discussions. We had talked about death in general, but to sit and look into the eyes of someone that you love dearly. . . and to talk about your own finality is something quite different. It was difficult for my dad to talk on that level. He was so much like Joe. I never realized it until that day. I saw it more each and every day that he stayed with me. Dad promised me that there would be no funeral and that he would donate my body to cancer research. "I found out they don't want my organs," I said. "I never knew you couldn't donate your organs if you had cancer. I can donate my eyes though. I'd like to donate them to someone so they can have a chance to see."

Every time Dad got tears in his eyes, I would say, "Dad, you promised! Dad, please be happy." It broke my heart when I thought about how much I wanted the pain to be over; not just for me but for everyone in my life.

"And one more thing, Dad. If they tell you that I'm not going to make it through the night, I don't want to know. Don't tell me." I hesitated for a moment. "You know, on second thought, I do want to know. If they tell you I'm not going to make it, you let me know because I'm going to get the longest extension cord I can find. I'm going to plug it into my phone and I'm going to call every person I know. I'm going to walk up and down those halls and I'm not going to stop. I figure as long as you're walking and talking, you ain't gonna die," I said.

We arrived at my doctors office to discover that he had been trying to reach me. All my tests had come back inconclusive, yet he had placed a phone call to the doctor at Metro University Medical Center - a bone marrow transplant center. Dr. Douglas discussed my case with him in great detail. The transplant specialist felt sure that I was relapsing and wanted to do a transplant as soon as possible.

Since my blood counts were so low, Doctor Douglas sent me to the oncology unit to receive multiple transfusions. I felt as though I was walking toward my execution. I began to cry. "I can't believe I'm back here. I have leukemia again," I thought. I took a deep breath as my path met the arms that embraced me. Each of the nurses had tears in their eyes. They gave me a hug and said, "I'm so sorry."

I attempted to smile, although my body was shaking throughout. "I'm back," I said. Somehow I felt relieved. There was nothing more to fight.

It felt good to give someone else the primary responsibility for taking care of me. I knew that it was my responsibility to take care of myself, but at least I had someone helping me. I knew those people loved me. It was the only place that I could fall apart and have someone catch me. They wanted so much for me to live. They didn't have any expectations of me and they didn't want me to "be" anything for them. I could cry when I was depressed. I could get angry when I didn't feel good. They understood. They were just thankful that I was alive.

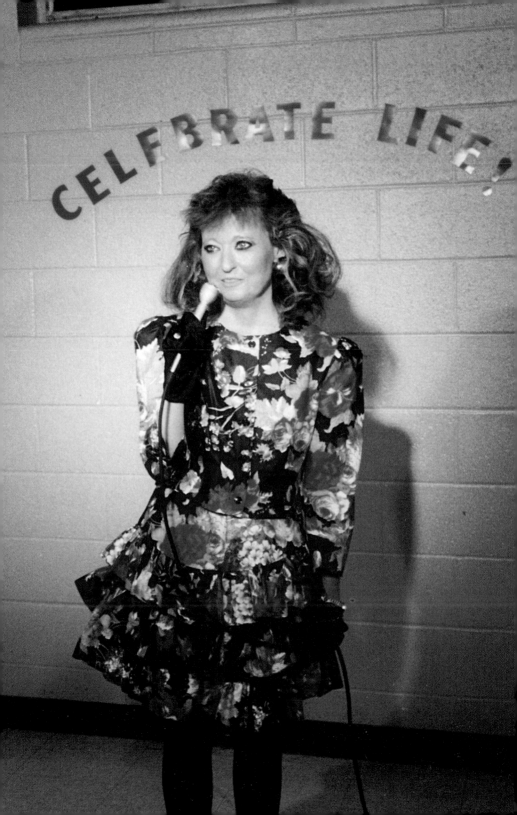

# Celebrate Life
## *is dedicated to*

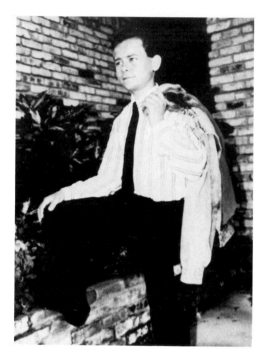

# *Ashley Bradford*
### *who lost his battle to Leukemia*
### *while searching for a donor*
### *Born:  January 22, 1976*
### *Died:  October 11, 1990*

# PART III

# CELEBRATE LIFE

## In the Words of Ashley Bradford before his death:

## TO THOSE I LOVE AND TO THOSE WHO LOVE ME

When I am gone, release me, let me go
I have so many things to see and so
You musn't tie yourself to me with tears
Be happy that we had so many years

I gave you my love. You can only guess
How much you gave me in happiness
I thank you for the love you each have shown
But now it's time I traveled on alone

So grieve a while for me, if grieve you must
Then let your grief be comforted by trust
It's only for a while that we must part
So bless the memories within your heart.

I won't be far away, for life goes on
So if you need me, call and I will come
Though you can't see me or touch me
I'll be near and if you listen with all
   your heart, you'll find
All my love around you soft and clear

And then, when you must come this way alone,
I'll greet you with a smile and say, "Welcome Home."

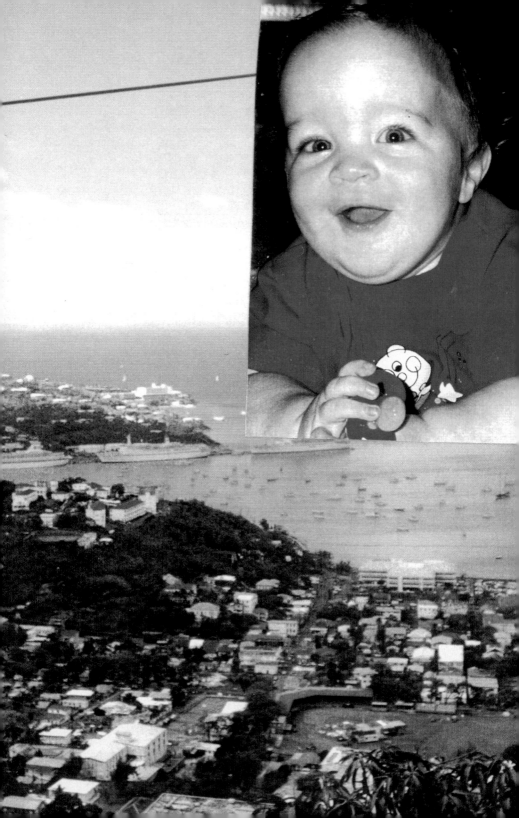

# CHAPTER ONE

## The Start of a Miracle

The next morning, I was in Dr. Mitchell's office with my Dad to discuss options for treatment. We knew the chances of finding a donor were very slim.

"If we could find an unrelated donor that was a perfect match for you, which may be possible since you have a fairly common tissue type, your chance of being completely cured this time is about 95%," he said.

I wanted to run away. I kept thinking about a man who called me while I was in the hospital the first time. He had told me that whatever I read about leukemia research was already out of date. "That's how fast they are progressing in treatment," he said. Surely there was some place I could go and have some other form of treatment done. I talked to Dr. Douglas about wanting to go somewhere else. I didn't tell him why. But he knew.

"If you were some 'schmuck' who I didn't care about I would say, "Go ahead. I've given you what I believe to be the best advise as your oncologist, but you have a right to make your decision. But with you, I will do everything in my power to keep you from going," he said.

In my heart I knew what I had to do. I knew I would end up having the transplant. I called other treatment centers that had the latest "experimental" treatments. They were having good results. The problem was that they just didn't return phone calls. Each day I tried to escape from my fate: I would see the faces of the children that appeared to me just a few nights before. I heard their voices say, "Please fight for us."

I heard another voice say: "Christine, we have a treatment that is guaranteed to cure you. You can have as many children as you want. The only drawback is all those children that need a transplant will die because you will not understand the depth of their need." After hearing that voice, I knew what my choice would be.

I remembered the words that God had spoken to me on my staircase. "The choice is yours. You are the master of your destiny. It has been that way from the beginning." I thought "holding on" meant fighting with everything inside of me. I didn't know it meant to trust. God has given us the ability within ourselves to survive, but I think there comes a time when "the battle to survive" becomes our worst enemy. We need to have faith that no matter what comes our way there is a power greater than ourselves that can and *will* provide in our best interest.

The next morning I called Dr. Mitchell and told him to start the search for a donor. At Dr. Douglas's insistence I activated the bone marrow computer registry earlier that year. The registry is a database of individuals that have agreed to donate their bone marrow if ever needed. Dr. Mitchell asked me to come in to the lab so they could draw some blood to begin the search.

He told me that I would need to have a round of chemotherapy in an attempt to get me into a second remission. I would need to have a donor by that time since the remission would only last a few months at the longest. Because the odds were so slim that I would find a donor, I started my own "bone marrow drive" and community awareness campaign. I designed a flier that had a brief synopsis of my life, statistics were given concerning the need for donors, and a brief explanation of the procedure of donating. I called several people and got them to serve as coordinators of my drive in their areas. The support I received was overwhelming.

Churches and businesses were coordinating efforts for people to be tested as potential donors. My church had a bone marrow drive in my behalf. Hundreds of individuals were donating blood. So many people were trying to find the "needle in my haystack" - a donor. At the time I began looking for a donor there were 61,000 in the National Bone Marrow Registry. That was in December of 1989. The search in the National Bone Marrow Registry turned up nothing.

After only three days of treatment all signs of leukemia has disappeared. I was told that it would take approximately one month for a remission to occur. Although I didn't have a biopsy, it appeared that my marrow had been purged of any cancer cells in just a few days.

I spent my days listening to modern Christian music at the highest decibel that the headphone speakers would allow. There were three songs I played continuously. They were upbeat and each lyric spoke of the struggle for survival. I allowed the music to permeate my entire being.

When I wasn't listening to music, I was calling people in an attempt to get more individuals listed in the registry. The following day was New Year's Eve. I knew that at midnight the statistic would be the same. Approximately 10,000 lives had been lost that year because they could not find a donor for the transplant they needed to save their life.

I thought about the tragedy of wasted lives. There were so many people that deserved a chance to live and they could have it if they could just find their missing puzzle piece. I wanted 1990 to be different; not just for me but for everyone that had suffered the tragedy of being diagnosed with cancer. "There is no reason why anyone should have to die of Leukemia anymore," I thought to myself.

The following day my Dad paid to access all of the international registries. The Anthony Nolan registry in London, England was included. To everybody's shock and amazement, three potentially perfect matches were found. Each of them would have to be contacted to give a blood sample. Their blood would be mixed with mine to determine if the blood was compatible.
It usually takes months, if ever, to find a person that partially matches the patient's tissue type. There are three combinations of antigens that must match before a person can be a donor. So often the patient will gain hope because one potential match will be found. The person will match one set of antigens. But frequently, the second series of testing determines that the tissue type is different. The patient must begin the search again. Meanwhile, the patient is becoming weaker and more ill. Often they die in the process. That is why we are losing so many lives to ieukemia.

All three of my potential donors had already passed the first two tests. They were contacted and within one week each of them had blood drawn for the final testing. I received a phone call from Metro University Medical Center: The blood from each potential donor was on its way to the states.

Dr.Douglas came running into my room as if he had heard there were an emergency. He looked at me and knew that I had been crying.

"They told you," he said. He looked so disappointed. As I looked into his eyes he said, "I wanted to be the one to tell you."

I said, "Douglas, you know the chance of that happening...The chance of finding one donor. . ."

Everyone involved knew what a miracle had happened. The chance of finding one donor is astonishing. But having three is extraordinary.

Two weeks later, the medical staff had chosen a perfect match for my bone marrow transplant. It was a male. All I knew was his name was John F. and he was from Scotland. The transplant was set for March 30, 1990.

I have heard many oncologists say the most difficult phenomenon known to mankind is to get through a bone marrow transplant from an unrelated donor. As I look back on my experience, I believe that statement to be true. The treatment of chemotherapy for leukemia is never an easy one - you just try to make the best out of a bad situation. But it no way prepares you for the suffering of a bone marrow transplant.

My initial round of chemotherapy - which put me into a second remission - was filled with its own struggles. I put a huge monthly calendar on the wall as I had done each time I underwent a lengthy admission to the hospital. I would mark each day off with a "smiley face" sticker to count the days that I had gotten through. Each of those "smiley faces" meant I was one step closer to my goal.

As I was counting the days of my hospitalization prior to my transplant, my hemorrhaging intensified. I had been told repeatedly that the chemotherapy treatments would leave me sterile for a couple of years. But every month I continued to menstruate.

I would smile and think to myself, "Thank you, Jesus."

My blood counts always recovered quickly following treatment. After the high-dose chemotherapy I received prior to my transplant, the counts were much slower in returning to normal. I had been passing blood clots for weeks when, unexpectantly, the bleeding intensified. I checked my personal calendar. It was the day that I was to start my period. The delayed production of platelets coupled with the onset of my period set the stage for serious hemorrhaging. My doctor ordered a prescription for birth control pills to enable the bleeding to stop.

A nurse brought a birth control pill in with my other medications. All I could think about was how much I wanted a baby. I didn't want to do anything to jeopardize my chance of maintaining my fertility.

When my doctor came in to see me, I asked him, "Is it confrontation time?" He nodded in agreement although he looked as though he wanted to throw me out the window.

He smiled at me and said, "Tell me why you don't want to take the pill."

"Douglas, you know why," I said, "I know that it's not a probability. Everyone has told me that I will be sterile after the transplant, but I'm not sterile now. I just don't want to do anything to jeopardize that. You know how much I want a baby. If there is any possibility, just a *possibility*...that's good enough for me.

As he looked at me, I knew that he understood. He was the one that told me that I had leukemia when I was five-and-one-half months pregnant. He was with me when my baby died and he had to continue monitoring my chemotherapy during the 12 hours I spent in labor. I didn't have to say anything else.

"If you *promise* me that you will be honest and tell me if it gets any worse. . . I'm not talking about waiting until you're losing so much blood that we can't even transfuse you. . ." he said.

I didn't let him finish his sentence before I said, "I promise."

Within three days the bleeding stopped. I was no longer passing clots. It looked as though my prayer had been answered.

The following weekend I got up to go to the bathroom. It was then I realized I had begun bleeding again. I was alarmed as I thought about the consequences of my discovery. I wanted to hide so no one would find out. With each hour the clotting escalated. By evening I was passing approximately 20 blood clots an hour. Each clot was 3 to 4 inches in diameter.

I collapsed twice and could not pull myself up from the floor. I was told to stay in bed and to not get up for any reason. The nurses called my doctor. He was off-duty that weekend. His partner was making rounds. The nurses tattled and I was on a birth control pill by evening.

Dr. Douglas was on-duty the next day. As he walked into my room I said, "Well, I just gave birth to a racquetball."

He said, "Yeah, I heard. I also heard you keep falling asleep on the floor. Do you think there is any correlation between that and your bleeding?" Without allowing me to respond he said, "Ten out of ten women will stop menstruating with high-dose chemotherapy. You never have stopped. I would take that as a sign. If there is one thing that has become clear to me in the past two years, it is that nothing in **your** life happens by coincidence. It has got to be providential."

My doctor brought me back to reality as he did on so many occasions. He always presented the facts. Yet he always instilled in me the faith to believe that facts are facts until someone proves them to be different. We had many discussions about life and values. He believed in being responsible for your own health and using the resources available to you. He also knew that there was a power within each of us that went beyond our understanding.

I did a lot of thinking while I was at Dallas Community Hospital. I thought about Joe. I thought about my disease and how I was fighting with every thing inside of me to live. Joe was giving in to his disease. He wasn't experiencing the pain that I was experiencing. He anesthetized his pain.

As I laid in my hospital bed with toxic doses of chemotherapy running through my veins and having chills with an intensity equivalent to convulsions, I began to see Joe for what he really was. Joe was an addict.

Although it is true that addiction is a disease, it is a disease with a cure. It is cured by making a choice. And that decision must be made before the temptation ever arises. If an addict waits until the time that a decision must be made. . .it is too late.

I remember thinking, "Joe, you may be an addict, but so am I." My pain of not changing had become greater than my pain of changing. I had reached the bottom of my addiction. My addiction was destroying everything around me. It was obliterating my relationships. It had robbed me of any happiness in my present life and it was robbing me of my future.

That night I realized that all of the things I had accused Joe of was everything that I had within myself. Somehow I thought if I could fill the vacuum inside of Joe, then my own emptiness would disappear. The answer to the void was within my own heart. I had understood that in my mind, but now I was really feeling it. I didn't want my drug any longer. I wanted to be free.

As I was pondering these thoughts, my mother walked into my room. It was approximately 10:30 P.M..

I looked at her in shock and said, "What are you doing here?"

She said "I'm going to spend the night. I just felt like my little girl needed me." She walked over to my bed and gave me a kiss on the forehead. She put her hand to my face and said, "You feel warm", and took a washcloth from the tray and wet it. As all mothers do when their child has a fever, she wrung out the washcloth, folded it in accordion style and placed it on my forehead.

The look on my face must have been one of total astonishment. She looked at me and said, "I told you, little girl, you're not going to go through this by yourself. I love you." She then pulled two chairs together and sat down in one of them. She put her legs in the other chair. She then put her reading glasses on and glanced down at the television guide. "What's on tonight?" she asked. "Are there any good late movies?"

I don't think I ever answered her question. Emotionally, I was taken back in age to the last time I ever really felt her love. I was probably three years old. I was sick and running a high fever. She had given me a kiss and put a wet washcloth on my forehead. I was lying in her bed. We were watching As the World Turns. I had learned to write at a very young age. That day I wrote in my diary "Today I was sick. Mommy and me watched T.V. She gave me a kiss. I love her."

As I thought about that day during my childhood and as I looked at the woman from whom I had so desperately sought her love for so long, I literally felt a sensation travel through my body. It was similar to a low frequency electrical shock. It went from the top of my head to the bottom of my feet. All the emotional scars from the pain that I experienced with her were instantaneously healed. I knew that she loved me. She could no longer hurt me.

That day was a turning point in my life. I discovered that my mother really did love me. I learned to accept her for who she was and in turn she accepted me. I laughed as I thought to myself, "My whole life is falling apart. I'm losing everything a person could possibly lose in this life and I'm finding everything that I have ever wanted."

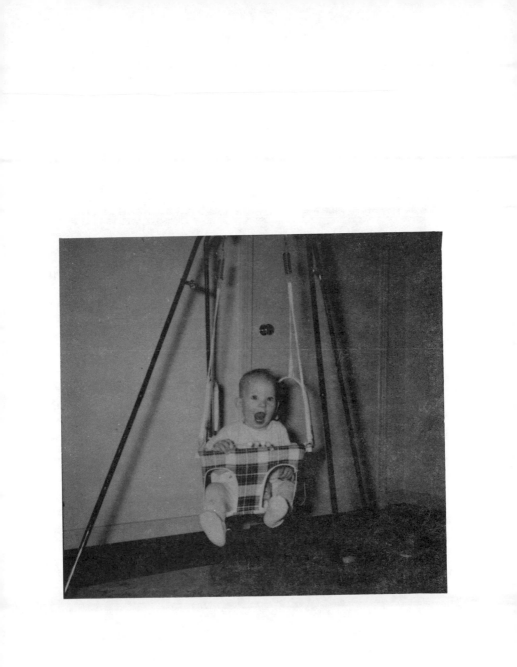

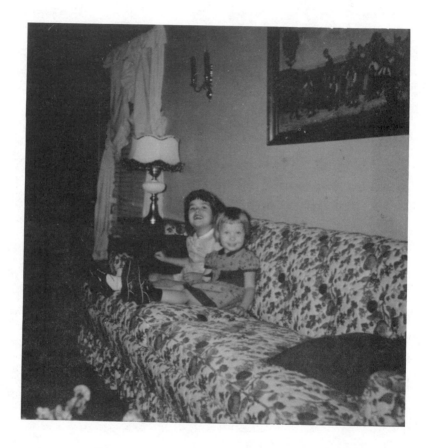

# CHAPTER TWO

## Awaiting the Transplant

Since my transplant was not scheduled until March 30, I spent the month prior to my hospital admission living life to its fullest. I was determined to not waste one minute of whatever life I had left.

Whenever I thought about the possibility of death, I would look in the mirror and think, "It just doesn't make sense. I don't look like a dying person. I don't feel like a dying person." I would take a long look into my eyes and look at the Christine that I knew lived deep within me. I thought, "Today. . .I am alive. My heart is still beating. I'm still breathing. That's what determines life. It has nothing to do with cancer."

I knew my recovery process was going to be extremely long and I would be in virtual isolation for approximately one year. With that knowledge, I wanted to put as much "living" as possible in to that short time period. I had lunch with different friends every day. I went dancing on weekends. I went to parties. I talked to everyone that I could about the need for bone marrow donors. I called organizations in an attempt to set-up bone marrow drives before I would enter my long hospital stay.

A few days before I went into the hospital, I tried one last time to contact my attorney. I had not called earlier because I did not want to squander any energy toward the negative forces within my life. I picked up the phone to dial the number. I was holding a copy of the letter my attorney had sent Joe on December 4, 1989. As I was waiting for the receptionist to answer - I read, "By your executing this waiver and returning it to me, my client will be able to go to court at her discretion anytime after the petition has been on file for sixty (60) days. She has requested that you do this and do not appear in court due to her health conditions."

I hung up the phone while I thought about the many months I spent holding on to Joe. Joe had walked out of my life exactly seven months to the day. Without my knowledge, Debra had called Joe when I relapsed. He was not home. She left him a message and told him that my leukemia had returned. She did not tell me she had done that until much later. She had been the only person Joe would talk to. Now he would no longer talk to her. He left his answering machine on and would not return her phone calls.

I again picked up the phone to call my attorney. He was not in the office. I talked with his partner. She was my age and was compassionate concerning the struggle I was experiencing.

I said, "Tami, I feel confident in my gut that somehow I'm going to be okay. I know a large part of that had to do with having the courage to look within. I look within and I see love. I don't want a divorce. I cannot honestly say that I want to end my marriage. I chose to marry Joe. I just didn't know some of the things that I know now. If I had known those things, I would have never married Joe. I loved him immensely. But I just didn't know."

She asked me to elaborate on what I was saying. I told her about the first time Joe asked me to marry him. "Tami, I told him I loved him but there were two things in my life that were not negotiable. I desperately wanted a baby. Joe has three children from his previous marriage. He had a vasectomy before we met.

He told me that he would have the vasectomy reversed. One month after our marriage I found out I was pregnant. Tami, I had never been happier in my life. Joe wrote me a letter and said he left because he couldn't give me what I wanted most in life. . .a child.

Tami, I found out Joe never had the vasectomy reversed. Apparently the vasectomy had come untied. His doctor did not want to sever the strings completely due to Joe's age; he might change his mind later. So. . his doctor tied them. After we lost the baby, while I was in the hospital, he actually had a complete vasectomy done. During our entire marriage, he never let me know. He just kept postponing the time that we would try and conceive.

We also had many discussions about values and lifestyle. Joe and I talked a lot about drugs since I was in the profession of human resource management. Then I found out he was using cocaine the night we announced our engagement. Tami, he lied to me. I cannot bring a suit against him because of conflict of personalities. It's so much more than that."

Tami said, "Let me ask you something. Knowing what you know now, would you have married Joe?"

With tears in my eyes I replied, "No way."

"Did you know that is grounds for annulment?" she asked.

"Annulment? How do you get an annulment when you've been married this length of time and have had a baby?" I asked.

"There are different grounds for annulment just like there are for divorce," she said. "It sounds to me like Joe induced you to marry him based on fraud. That is a misrepresentation of who and what he was," she said. "Have you lived with him since you found this out?"

"No. I found out all of it after he moved out." I told her. I turned my case over to Tami. She stopped proceedings for divorce and filed an amended petition for annulment based on fraud. The petition was mailed to Joe by certified mail on March 15, 1990.

The week before my transplant was scheduled, I was admitted to the cancer center at the hospital. The entire time I was there, I felt so unattractive. My entire self-esteem had always been based on what others thought. I was extremely self-conscious. I felt as though the people passing by were thinking, "Oh, God. . .I wonder what's wrong with her?" I was so frightened, that if anyone saw me without my wig and makeup, they wouldn't like me. If I had any advance warning that I was going to be taken somewhere, I tried to quickly put on some makeup. I always put on my wig in hopes that everyone would think it was my real hair. Of course, most of my limited excursions were for tests for some complication that had occurred. I consistently heard the same comment. . . "Honey, you need to leave your wig here. And those earrings need to stay." Although I never got away with my feeble attempt to cover my feelings of insecurity, I never stopped trying.

A nurse at Metro Medical Center, who is now a good friend of mine, loves to tell people about my at-tempts to play "dress up". She tells everyone about the numerous occasions she would enter my room to find my mascara and mirror in hand. I would be medicated to the point of intoxication. Janet tells the story. . . "and there she was with this mascara trying to put it on. And that lipstick! That lipstick would be down on her chin. You should have seen those earrings. She would always have a pair of earrings to match each nightgown that she had. . . like someone was going to see her."

One of the most difficult adjustments to having cancer, is being stripped of all defense mechanisms. A cancer patient does not get to choose when to become vulnerable; they are made vulnerable immediately upon diagnosis. We are not provided an opportunity to test the water to assure that it is safe before entering. A person that is told, "You have cancer" becomes a victim within themselves. To be victimized without a reserve of self-worth makes the battle of survival the most difficult thing to overcome. It is much like being thrown into cold water without having the knowledge to swim. Even though nature has given us all we need to survive, all too often we drown.

I believed with everything inside of me that it was possible for me to survive my bone marrow transplant. What I lacked was the confidence to believe that I was **going** to survive. There is a vast difference in believing that something is possible and believing that something is going to happen.

The elevator door opened. I heard the nurse say, "Well, here we are." I looked up to see a sign: "Bone Marrow Intensive Care Unit". There was nothing about the place that resembled a normal hospital wing. There was a nurse's station on one side of the unit with eight doors facing it. Each room had a small window in which the patients could be monitored. The window was extremely small. It was about 20 inches by 12 inches. It was just large enough for a nurse to see inside the patient's room.

The nurse opened the door to the room that was going to be my home for an indefinite time period. I took a deep breath. I had toured the facility earlier, yet I was flabbergasted when I was wheeled into the room. The room was approximately 8 feet by 10 feet. There was a small window in a far corner. It was offset from the rest of the room. The room reminded me of a prison cell.

I remember thinking, "God, how am I going to get through this? I can't even see outside." Each time I had a negative thought, my baby's face would come to mind. I continued to hear the words, "I love you, Mommy, please don't give up. Please fight for us."

Each intensive care room contained a special filtering system called a "HEPA" filter, which removed the germs in the air that could cause infection. For the system to be effective, the door had to be closed as much as possible. No one except my parents and the bone marrow transplant staff were allowed to enter my room and I was not allowed to leave. For 12 weeks, that germ-free cubicle was my home. It was then that I realized the seriousness of the disease of leukemia. Everyone who entered the room had to wash their hands before entering. They were required to wear sterile masks and gloves. My parents came to the hospital every day. The visitation hours were restricted, but my parents stayed by my side every moment that was allowed.

I was used to the chemotherapy I would receive, but the radiation treatments were a new experience. The treatments were scheduled, so I knew exactly what time I would need to be ready. I remember frantically trying to apply my makeup. I brushed out my wig and put a new bright colored bow in it. Before I could finish "getting ready", I was stopped in my process. Not only was I told that I could not wear my wig, but I had to remove my makeup. Feeling totally humiliated, I strolled over to the sink with my two IV poles and washed my face. I scowled with an expression of hatred toward the person who had the audacity to tell me to take my makeup off. I dried my face with a towel, turned around and walked toward the door. A stretcher was waiting for me.

The radiologist strategically positioned my stretcher in the corner of a very large room. I was strapped to the table to prevent my body from moving during the treatment. The radiology staff left me in total isolation as they exited to a glass protected room from which they would speak to me through a microphone.

I inspected the area around me. I looked at my body that was strapped down on the stretcher. I felt totally defenseless. I thought, "This is great. The treatment is so pernocuous that it's not safe for human consumption. Everyone that knows anything about this "stuff" has run for protection." The lack of human touch was debilitating. I felt as though I was in an execution chamber while everyone watched me struggle for my last breath. There was no one to stand by me and hold my hand. I was totally alone. Everyone was in their safe protected environment while the radiation was having a "free-for-all" with my body.

It seemed as though hours had passed since I had heard anything from that "little glass room". I thought, "Now, what if everyone has left me strapped to this table and they're not going to come back and get me?" As I thought about that possibility, I began to laugh. I thought, "I would love to do this to someone; strap them down, enter my shielded glass room and not come back. I would love to watch people's reaction." I wondered how many people would lie there for hours without question. They would never get up until the appropriate "authority" figure gave them permission.
The thoughts that go through a cancer patient's mind are incredible. It is a constant battle between passivity and activity. But one that becomes a vague memory with time.

My transplant was scheduled for March 30, 1990 at 12:30 A.M.. A doctor from Wales was bringing the donated marrow to Dallas. Dr. Mitchell went to the airport to meet him. It was 1:00 A.M. when Dr. Mitchell arrived at the hospital. It was storming on that night. The roads were slick and the news on television was reporting many accidents. My dad said, "I can just see getting that marrow all the way to Dallas from Scotland and then Mitchell has a wreck on the way to the hospital."

I said, "That's okay. They would bring him to Metro Medical anyway. It would just get here faster. He would be in an ambulance."

At that moment, Dr. Mitchell stuck his head in to my room. In his hand was the handle of a styrofoam ice chest. "We got it," he said. His tie was loosened. His sleeves were pushed up. He looked like he was "off-duty" and had picked up a six-pack of beer that was being iced down in a cooler. But I knew that inside that ice chest was the key to my survival.

I looked at my parents. They had been sitting by my bed throughout the day. The social worker arranged for them to stay in the hospital hotel, but they wanted to be with me during the transplant procedure. We all looked at each other with fear in our eyes, afraid to say anything that might reflect our true inner thoughts.

I looked at the clock. My heart started palpitating. The stakes were exorbitant. The transplant determined whether I would live or die. It was "winner takes all." As I laid on my hospital bed, I tried to preserve the image of my son. I fostered the remembrance of the children that said, "Please fight for us. We can't fight for ourselves." I focused on each of their faces; I looked deeply into their eyes. It gave me strength to hold on.

Although I did not know any of the patients on the unit, my parents had gotten to know each of their families extremely well. Mom and Dad would often buy donuts and coffee for everybody, and they would all sit and chat as they waited to see loved ones. I glanced at the wall behind my bed. I thought about the patient in the next room. I did not know who it was but I knew being on the unit they were afraid. It did not matter what age they were. The transplant center was for adults. But within each of us was a frightened child.

I asked my mother, "Mom, tell me about the people that are in here. Who else is having a transplant?"

She told me about each person on the unit. She started with the person at the very end of the hall. She told me her name, age, marital status, and where she was from. She talked about the family members that were with her. She would describe to me the type of cancer that she had and if she had her transplant yet. She would then tell me if she had an unrelated donor, a sibling donor or if she was using her own marrow. Then she would describe the person in the next room with the same detail.

As she spoke, I would mentally take my baby in my arms and picture myself entering their room. I would stand quietly where the patient could not see me or hear me. I would recapitulate how special the person was and how much they were loved. If during my visualization, I saw that the patient was asleep, I would walk over to their bed and pray with them. I mentally put my baby in the bed with them. I said, "This is my strength and he is the reason that I am choosing to go on. I know that there is a desire deep within your heart. Look within yourself and discover what that desire is and don't ever let go." I visualized myself going from room to room. I was standing in the hallway when the nurse opened the door to my hospital room. I safely tucked my son away in my heart and slipped into bed.

"Were you asleep?" the nurse asked.

"Well, we are all ready. This is your marrow," she said.

"So, that's marrow?" Dad said as he stood up and took off his glasses. He wanted to get a closer look. I could tell he was just as fascinated as I was. I looked at the clock. It was 1:30 A.M..

"It looks like blood," I said. I was amazed at the composition. "It looks a lot like platelets."

"Now, how does this work?" Dad asked.

It's funny - we were given educational literature and viewed films about bone marrow transplantation. Yet, each of us acted like we never heard a word that anyone had spoken to us. For some reason when it is the marrow for *your* transplant you become void of any knowledge that should have prepared you for the process.

The nurse stood on her tip-toes to hang the bag of marrow on the IV pole. I had approximately four other medications and liquids running through my catheter simultaneously.  She turned and looked at Dad. "Well, it's real easy," she said. "We just hang it on the pole like I just did. And then I hook it up to one of the ports in her central line (catheter) and it's ready to go."

Dad was standing over my bed looking at the marrow and watching the nurse start the procedure. He was mystified by the paradox of complexity and simplici- ty. "So it's just like a transfusion?" Dad asked.

"Pretty much," she replied. "It goes right through the vein and travels into the bloodstream."

"Well, how does it know where to go?" Dad asked.

Watching Dad be fascinated by the transplant reminded me of myself as a child. I was notorious for asking questions such as "Daddy, where did God come from?" I continued to observe my dad as he scrutinized everything that the nurse was doing.

I reached out and touched the nurse on her arm. I said, "You know, you can make up anything you want. We wouldn't know the difference."

She laughed and said, "It's okay. No one can really answer that one. We just know that it works. It somehow finds it's way to the bone which is the foundation of the actual marrow. It makes a new home for itself and starts to do what it is supposed to do which is manufacture blood cells."

The transplant began at 1:30 A.M.. At 3:30 A.M., my parents went to the hotel in the next building. The procedure was completed at 7:30 A.M. the following morning.

Dr. Mitchell arrived early the next morning. As he walked in, I said "*That* was a transplant? That was a piece of cake." My doctor explained to me that it would take about two weeks before we knew if the transplant was a success. A graft would take place and, if successful, my body would take on my donor's marrow. I would begin to manufacture *his* blood cells.

But he cautioned me, "Christine, the next few weeks will be extremely dangerous. You will be vulnerable to every disease, virus, bacteria and infection known to man. And we'll need to watch for Graft-Versus-Host Disease, which is the rejection of the transplanted marrow. I was totally dependent on synthetic drugs and antibiotics to keep me alive. Every natural fighter cell that I was born with had been destroyed. I had no marrow and I was no longer manufacturing my own blood cells. I received multiple transfusions daily.

Each day I watched the antibiotics enter my blood stream through the central line catheter. I used guided imagery principles to visualize all of the bacteria, viruses or infections being destroyed as the medication traveled throughout my body.

I visualized the drugs traveling past my ovaries. By closing my eyes I could paint a picture in my mind of my ovaries being protected by a thick wall. Any time that the chemotherapy or radiation attempted to damage my ovaries, I would picture my ovum uniting together.

I also would mentally picture my new marrow making friends with my bone structure. I visualized the marrow unpacking and decorating it's new home. Since my donor was from Scotland, everything that the marrow brought in was plaid. The marrow began to build a blood manufacturing plant. In my mind the plant resembled a paint manufacturing company. It was equipped with an assembly line, security guards, carpenters and painters. I imagined the red blood cells being mixed in a huge tank.

Whoever entered my room for a specific purpose would be assigned a role. I would dress them in the appropriate attire and give them the tools they needed to accomplish their job effectively. The nurse that administered the kidney function test once a week had no idea that in my mind she was wearing overalls and a hard hat. In reality, she gave me a shot to send a tracer through my system to mark the kidney levels. In my mind, however, the needle was a nail. It was her job to hammer sheet metal around my kidneys to keep them protected from any damage that the transplant could cause.

"Whatever the mind can conceive and believe, the body can achieve." Everything in my immune system had been destroyed. It became apparent to me that the immune system is not where the battle of cancer is fought. If it is not where the battle is fought, neither is it where the battle is won.

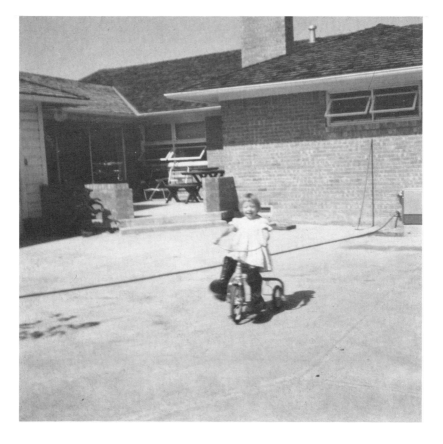

Dr. Douglas and his wife came to visit me during that week. I remember telling him, "Man, I've never felt so good in all of my life. This transplant stuff is a 'piece of cake.'" I was sitting-up in bed behaving as "Miss Congeniality" while in actuality I was intoxicated from the dilaudid. I felt as though I was floating around the room.

A nurse that I knew well suspected that I was not completely coherent. She entered my room one afternoon and asked me, "Christine, are you okay? Are you getting too much of this stuff?"

I assured her that I was fine. I said, "No, it's really helping. I feel a lot better. My mouth is still sore but it doesn't hurt like it did." I couldn't even feel my mouth.

Not believing me she consulted with another nurse. "How much Dilaudid is Christine getting? Is she on too much? She just seems so happy." The other nurse laughed and said, "She's fine. Christine is always like that."

I think my charade could have continued indefinitely if I would have been more selective about disclosing my new-found knowledge. It was a Thursday morning. A nurse came in to help me with a shower. I informed her that I wanted to take a bath, but she needed to call housekeeping first. "There are dead birds in my bathtub. Somebody needs to get them out," I said.

My parents arrived at that time. The nurse told them that she was going to call housekeeping to remove the birds from my bathtub. She left the room and I said, "She's such a sweet-heart. You know, last night there was a cow in there. I had already taken my bath so he wasn't in my way."

About that time, I found myself being interrogated several times a day. I would be asked questions like, "What is your name? Where do you live?" I think it was the question, "Do you know what hospital you are in?" that got me into trouble. I replied, "Well, of course, I'm in General Hospital." The next thing I knew my self-regulating pump was taken away and a slow drip bottle of dilaudid was ordered instead. The dosage was drastically decreased.

As I had done every month since delivery of the baby, I started my period. The medical staff was shocked. I was placed on an excessive dose of hormones to curtail the bleeding. Everytime I had to swallow the hormones, I cried improvidently.

My blood pressure had been slowly increasing. I was experiencing blinding headaches. The medical staff felt sure I was experiencing withdrawals from the narcotic. I felt sure that if they would just give my dilaudid back - I would be fine. The pain was back. But, in reality I knew it had never left. One day I would have to face it again. And then - there would be no turning back.

It was a Friday night when my tolerance reached its maximum limitation. I could not stand to move my head one inch without screaming in pain. I did not get any sleep that night. The nursing staff was in my room every 10 minutes trying to find something to alleviate the pain. Dr. Mitchell was called into the hospital to examine me.

"We're going to find out what's causing this and get to the bottom of it," he said. There were many times that he would reach out to me and be my only ray of hope. I would often feel him going beyond his professional obligations of providing medical care and expertise. The concern came from his heart. I could feel the genuine compassion from the personal relationship we had established. It was often that personal touch that got me through the day.

It was approximately 4:00 A.M. when I got out of bed to go to the bathroom. I pushed the two IV poles in front of me. On that particular night, I never made it past the entrance of the bathroom door. I began to turn around and fell to the floor. I hit my head on the edge of the toilet seat. The IV pole tilted as if it was going to fall on top of me. I tried to protect my body from what appeared was going to be an inevitable crash. I couldn't move. I looked out of the corner of my eye. I could see the pole balancing itself as it rocked back and forth.

Approximately 18 inches from my reach was the emergency call button. I tried to focus my eyes on it, but everything in the room was blurred. I reached up to pull the chain, which was attached to the button. I couldn't lift my arms from the floor. After several attempts, I knew I was in serious trouble. I tried to yell for help. The sound of my voice was no louder than a whisper. My entire body shook as I tried to make contact with the emergency button. The button might as well have been on the other side of the room. My body was sprawled in the small area between the door and the toilet. The left side of my face was pressed against the floor. I could not lift my head. No one could see that I had fallen. I closed my eyes and gathered every bit of strength that I could muster within me.

"Help Me-e-e," I uttered. The cry for help sounded much like a groan. After several attempts of calling out, I felt my chest collapse to the floor. I opened my eyes and whispered to myself, "God help me." Within a few minutes I heard my hospital door open. I opened my eyes.

"Christine?" I heard a voice call out. It was the nurse on duty. He walked to the partially opened door and said, "Oh, my God! Christine, are you okay?"

I told him that I could not move. He pushed the emergency button. Several nurses ran in to help. I don't remember what happened after that. Somehow I got back in bed and was back on a high dose of dilaudid. The pain was still extreme but at least it was no longer insufferable.

Early the following morning I was taken to X-ray for multiple tests. The medical staff felt sure that I was hemorrhaging from the brain. My parents arrived early that morning. My mother asked about the implications if I were, in fact, hemorrhaging. She was told they would have to drill a hole in my head to drain the blood. Before the results were back, she asked my doctor about that procedure. He informed her that it would be impossible to drill a hole in my head. If they did, I would bleed to death.

"She has no platelets," he said.

Once again, I was in a no-win situation. For the first time since I had gotten sick - I got angry. I felt like I was being punished. I cried to my parents that day. "It's not fair," I said. "I feel like I'm being punished. I haven't done anything wrong!" I told God that I would do anything to live. I accepted that I would never be able to have children. I agreed to go through the transplant process and use it to help others. But I had been through enough ... This was not part of the bargain.

I think if it had not been for a technician adminis-tering the MRI and CAT-scans, I don't think I would have made it through the tests. One of my nurses went down with me on the elevator and held my hand until the tests began. I was being taken back to my room, as I over-heard my doctor ask the nurse that took me down for tests, how the tests went.

"I'm pretty sure I saw blood on the brain," she said. "But, of course, I wasn't allowed in there so - I don't know."

My doctor immediately called the Imaging Center. I was definitely hemorrhaging from the brain and bleeding profusely. The normal procedure was to drill a small hole in my head and allow the blood to drain but in my case, that option was impossible. A neurologist was called immediately. He asked me the same questions he had asked last week. I thought I was doing well until I was later told that we had a new president: George Washington.

Each day the tests would continue, but the pain was not getting any better and the hemorrhaging got worse. The neurologist was once again called to my room. My body was languid. All I could do was gaze into space. I could feel death all around me.

The neurologist said, "I heard you're not having a very good day."

I smiled at him and said, "No, I'm not but it could always be worse". He commented to me about my remarkable attitude.

He said, "Well, I've been told that you are a pretty special person around here. And Dr. Mitchell is going to personally hold me responsible unless we get this under control so. . . that's what we're going to do."

"Christine, we need for the brain to absorb the blood. Since you don't have any platelets, that is really your only alternative. Now, in order for that to happen, you need to be totally still. I'm going to put your bed down flat. I don't want you to use a pillow. The head must remain flat at all times. Try not to move at all. I'll have the nurses pull the monitor window blinds so the light from the hall will not shine in here."

For 10 days I laid in total darkness. I could not have any lights on. The television and radio had to remain off. The switchboard routed my phone calls so the phone would not ring in my room. I was not allowed to talk. Any oral medications were given to me with a straw since I was prohibited from lifting my head. My bed was only permitted to be raised 10 degrees and that was for limited time periods every other day. I could not get up to go to the bathroom.

After a couple of days, I began to experience a deep depression. I withdrew into a "blue funk" that I could not overcome. Each day I became more despondent. My parents tried to encourage me. I could only lay there. The word had gotten out that I was not doing well. I received cards and letters from friends saying, "Christine, please don't give up. We need you down here. Please fight." My parents would read the sentiments to me. But, for the first time in my life, I didn't care if I lived or died. I told my parents that I didn't want them to say anything else.

My doctor knew I had become severely depressed. I think my hopelessness frightened everyone more than any medical complication could have ever done. No one had ever seen me so low. Most people had never seen me without a smile; even during the roughest of times. People who were close to me would drop by the hospital. Dr. Mitchell told the nurses to let them in if I wanted to see them. I refused. I didn't want to see anyone.

One day I was imagining what it was like to die. I was pondering the instantaneous conversion from life to death; that second that we are changed in the twinkling of an eye. . . a second. It was always that "second" that kept me going. I wasn't afraid of being dead. I believe in Heaven. It was really the desire of my heart to live with Jesus one day. And it wasn't dying that I feared. I had been to death's door many times. It was that second; going from the known to the unknown.

As I was meditating on that thought, my door opened. It was my friend Debra. "Hey, gal," she said as her voice cracked. She reached over and stroked my face. I tried not to look at her.

"You know, girl, you just gotta pull through this because everyone loves you and we're all praying for ya," she said. I could see out of the corner of my eye that she was crying.

"So you're not gonna look at me?" she asked.

I turned my head and her eyes were red from crying. She had so much love in her heart for me. I loved her immensely. Debra was my best friend at that time. She had stood by my side from the very first day that I met her. I was so angry with her for coming to the hospital when I was ready to die. As our eyes looked deep into the soul of the other, the bond that we had developed was penetrating the profundity of my being. I began to cry.

"Debra, I want to die," I said.

"Well, that's just too bad," she said "because we need you down here. Christine, you are so loved. You know, a bunch of us were talking last night after church and were praying for you. . .Desi started crying and said, "God, you can't let anything happen to her because we need her. I know that's selfish. But, God, we need her down here."

I just looked at her and cried. She was crying also. There was nothing more to say. That magic spirit of life, the gift of love, was saying it all. I had wrapped my life up into a neat little package and was waiting to die. Debra untied the package. She loved me with everything inside of her. No death could come between that. When I gave up. . . Debra took over. She refused to let me die.

Within 24 hours, my blood pressure was coming down. For nearly two weeks the nurses took my vital signs every 15 minutes. All vital signs were returning to normal. The pain was starting to subside. By the end of the week the brain had absorbed all the blood. I was no longer hemorrhaging. I was going to live.

Within three days, my entire world began to change. Dr. Mitchell made preparations to release me from the hospital. I experienced extreme anxiety thinking about not being in my protective environment any longer. The nursing staff was wonderful. It was as if they read my mind.

Before I was released from the hospital, I received physical therapy. After the brain hemorrhage, I was not allowed to move. I had been in bed for such a long time, that my muscles had atrophied. The physical therapist would come into my room and assist me in moving my legs and arms. Within a few days, I was able to pull myself up and put my feet on the floor. I could stand erect.

The therapist had tied me to herself with something that looked much like a karate belt. I was given a walker to keep from falling. The day came for me to take my first step. I discovered that although my brain had received the message, "Christine, let's start with one step. Put your left foot first," my brain would not send the message to my legs. I couldn't move. It was as though I had forgotten how to walk.

I thought, "My God, I can't walk." I looked at my therapist to see what her reaction was. As I had done with the doctor that had administered the neurology tests. . . .I lied. The same little girl that had always hidden when she was afraid, used the same defense mechanisms once again. I knew that if the therapist knew that I couldn't walk, I would not be allowed to go home. I looked at her and said, "I'm real tired. Can we walk tomorrow?" I put that big smile on my face as if everything was fine.

She grabbed my hand and said, "Sure, that's fine. You did good today."

As she was leaving the room, Dr. Mitchell was coming in. He wanted to keep me in the hospital another week to monitor the Graft vs. Host disease. I knew that many patients had contracted GVH. Some of them had experienced excessive complications and died. I became terrified that I was going to be the next one to go. A week earlier I had been ready. But now I wanted to live. My parents soon arrived.

"Hi, Sweet-heart," Dad said.

"Did the physical therapist come?" Mom asked.

I told them she had come in about an hour before. They knew how severely depressed I had become. My mother had tried to get me to go outside of my room. "Do you want to go for a ride?" she asked. "I'll get the wheelchair." I started to cry.

"I have Graft vs. Host Disease. Mitchell said I can't go home," I told them. "Am I going to die?"

"No, you're not going to die. Christine, everyone up here has Graft vs. Host. You're the only one who hasn't had it.

I was terrified I was going to be different. God had done so much for me. I kept thinking, "I didn't have the faith. God gave me a choice and I made my choice last week. I wanted to die." I was so afraid I had made the decision in my mind and now it was too late. My body was going to follow what it had been commanded to do. I had seen so many cancer patients give up. They became so afraid or tired - they did not want to go on.

Before I relapsed, I did seminars and workshops with cancer patients who had become clinically depressed. So often I saw it in their eyes. They truly believed they were going to die. Most often they did. I tried to remember the things I had shared with them.

I would often ask them, "When you close your eyes and visualize what your deepest fear is, what comes to mind?" The answer was always the same. . . death.

"So, what you are telling me is, that. . . maybe you're tired of fighting. You're scared because. . . why? Do you know?" I would ask.

Of course, the answer was always the same. "I don't want to die." Tears would flow. I would explain to them our minds cannot picture the words "can" and "can't," "do" or "don't." All it can see is what our subconscious mind tells it.

Patients would start their program with severe depression. Somewhere in the recovery process a release would take place. The laughter and play would be incredible. It was as if for the first time in their life, they were being allowed to play.

The rest of the seminar would be focused on the difference in saying, "I don't want to die" and saying "I want to live." The mind creates two totally different pictures. We would draw those pictures on paper, and literally burn the negative one in a trash can. They would then take the positive picture of life home with them. I told them to put it in a place where they could see it many times a day. It would serve as a constant reminder of their new thought patterns.

I wanted so much to burn the picture I had in my mind, but I was paralyzed with fear. All I knew is that I couldn't walk and I had Graft vs. Host disease. And a week earlier, I reached a point that I decided I did not want to live anymore.

While I was deep in thought, my mother had gone to get the wheelchair. She brought it into the room and said, "Let's go for a ride. Everyone wants to see you."

Somehow my mother talked me into going for a ride. I first had to put on matching gown, robe, socks and earrings, but I agreed to go. I put on some lipstick and my wig. I was shaking too badly to apply any other makeup successfully. I took a deep breath and put on my sterile mask and gloves. I swung my legs over to the side of the bed. My parents each grabbed an arm as they sat me down in the chair. I was terrified as they opened the door. My dad rolled the two IV poles attached to my body into the hallway. My mother followed, pushing me in the chair. Every face turned toward me.

"Well, lookie here. She's out!" I heard a nurse say.

"Hi Christine," another one said. "It's good to see you out. You look great."

Soon, all the family members came running toward me. "Christine, it's so nice to see you. I have heard so much about you. We love you, honey. We're praying for you." I was surrounded by faces and people and I had no idea who they were.

I wanted to go back to my room. I didn't know what I was "supposed" to do with these people. Everyone was watching me and smiling. I wanted to scream, "Mom, take me back," but I couldn't. All eyes were on me, so I kept smiling and continued to say, "It's so nice to meet you. Yes, I've heard Mom and Dad talk about you."

The first chance I got, I said in a very low voice where no one could hear me, "Take me back. I don't want to do this." My mother kept pushing the wheelchair.

"Hi Ron," she said. "I want you to meet Christine." I once again played my part. As he walked off, I gritted my teeth and said, "I want to go back. Take me back!" I dug my nails into my mother's hand that was pushing the wheel chair. I was trying to let her know how serious I was.

She quietly leaned over, smiled at the people that were passing by and gritted her teeth back at me. "Get your nails out of my hand or I'm going to take you down to the cafeteria." It was as if she was enjoying my pain. She rolled me through the double doors and took me to the office where a dear friend of mine worked. He was on the Board of Directors with me for Life-Link. He came out of his office to see me. And, as always. . .he made me laugh.

When Mom heard the laugh that she knew came from my heart, she wheeled me back to my room. That had been her goal. Upon arrival she asked, "Do you want to get back in bed?"

I said, "No. I want to sit up for a few minutes, but there is no room." There were only two chairs in the room and no space to walk around them.

Dad said, "I don't mind standing. It might do you some good to sit-up for a while, unless you're just really tired." They both lifted me out of the wheelchair and lowered me to the guest chair.

I looked behind the chair and began reading a "get well card" I had received. It was from a person whom I had never met. The person wrote that she had heard what had happened in my life and had been so touched by my faith. I wanted to laugh. I was petrified I was going to die because I didn't have any faith. I read on. Someone else whom I had never heard of had cancer. He wrote, "Your friends have talked about your courage and determination. It has given me something to hold on to." I then began to cry.

"Who are these people?" I asked.

Neither Mom or Dad knew the persons that had written the cards. Mom said "There's another one over here like that. Do you know Bill Johnson?" I didn't have any idea who he was. "He and his wife apparently lost a little boy to cancer. They wanted you to know they were praying for you."

Tears were streaming down my face. Each card I read was filled with words of encouragement and support. As I looked around the room, I felt like I had just woken up from the dead.

"Where did all these come from?" I asked.

There were cards taped everywhere. They were taped on all four walls, from the top of the wall by the ceiling, to the bottom of the wall by the floor. "They've been coming everyday for weeks. Your dad counted them and there are over 350 cards. You've got prayer-grams from churches all over the city. Your dad and I have been showing them to you, but you haven't really felt like looking at them."

As I looked around the room there was a huge banner that said, "We love you, Christine. It's not the same without you. Get well soon." There were balloon bouquets, pictures of friends and posters everywhere I looked. My eyes were drawn to the shelf that the television sat on. There were silk flower arrangements sitting on it. There was also an Easter basket and chocolate Easter bunny.

"Have we had Easter yet?" I asked.

"Honey, Easter was about three weeks ago," Dad said. "You don't remember Dr. Douglas and his wife coming to see you? They came a couple of times. They gave you the Easter bunny. It's Godiva chocolate." Godiva chocolate was my favorite.

"I want to read some of the cards. Will you help me?" I asked. Mom and Dad each took one of my arms and helped lift me out of the chair. It took every bit of strength I had to stand on my legs.

Dad got tears in his eyes. "Yeah, Sweetheart, you've had a lot of people praying for you. There's a lot of people who love you. You know, it was that way at Dallas Community Hospital, too, when you were looking for a donor. You had just as many cards. Half of them said they were going to give platelets and be listed in the registry. Do you remember that?" he asked. All I could do was cry.

"Bob, I think she has had enough for one day. She needs to get back in bed," Mom said. "Why don't you help her get in the wheelchair?"

"No!" I exclaimed. "I want to walk." It took me 20 minutes to take six steps but I felt like I had walked across Texas.

Hope you get well
soon.
  You see the lady with lots of
legs on the front of the card,
it's 'posed to make you
laugh.
    Love,
    Ryan KJ

# CHAPTER FOUR

## *The Glass Window*

I continued to have physical therapy for the next several days. Dressed with sterile masks, gloves and robe, I would take my walker through the hospital room door and start down the hall. At first, I couldn't make it past the room next door, but within days I was walking to the end of the hallway. I would stop when I reached the double doors that led out of the Bone Marrow Intensive-Care-Unit. I would peek through the small glass window in the door. Each day, I was one step closer to being able to walk out of that unit. I had seen the promised land. Nothing was going to stop me.

Dad was with me the day I was transferred out of ICU. He was taking the cards and letters down from the wall as the nurses were packing my bags. They were putting my possessions on a cart to be moved with me.

I closed my eyes and began to breathe deeply. I pictured in my mind the double doors that I had seen on my walks.

I opened my eyes to find all my walls bare and empty. There were four carts piled high with paraphanelia. A wheelchair was waiting to take me to my next destination. I hesitated for a moment as I brought myself back to reality. I had pictured myself walking - not riding - through the double doors. It was only a matter of seconds before I heard that inner voice say, "Yeah, but this way is so much faster."

I still had the picture in my mind when I heard a nurse's voice. She said, "Well, girl, are you ready?"

I smiled at the nurses who had become a special part of my life. "You betcha, I am!" I said. I jumped out of bed, sat in the wheelchair and took a deep breath. It was a breath of new life. The air filled the capacity of my lungs. It was filled with love and peace and joy. I had taken the breath of life. It was inside of me. I was free. I had *made* it through my transplant.

The week prior to my move out of the unit was the first time in my life I had ever said, "I quit." To reach the point that I truly would rather have died frightened me tremendously. During that time, however, I had thousands of individuals praying for me. I knew my life had changed the day Debra walked into my room. I found my miracle when I hit bottom and quit fighting so desperately to live. Paradoxically, it was when I "died to self" that I began to live. I spent my life trying to "die to self". That had been my prayer. I wanted to be every-thing that God wanted me to be. It was when I let go of the desire to "be". . . I "became." I became everything God wanted me to be. In actuality, I always had been because that is the way He made me. I just didn't know it.

I arrived in my new room much like a child who had been kept in a closet and not allowed to experience the beauty of life. When the nurse wheeled me through the door, I said, "My God, it's so big! And there's a window!" The room was not different than any other hospital room, but it just seemed that way.

The little child within me, the one that screamed for so long to be set free, was ecstatic to find her room filled with all the things she loved. I could watch the sun shine and the birds perch on the window sill. As I stood up from the wheelchair, I walked to the side of the bed where the window was. I could see grass and a tree. I remember thinking, "Oh, God, it's beautiful!" There were men working on the building across from my window.

A nurse walked in while I was looking out the window. "I'm sorry that you didn't get a better view," she said. "We can move you later if you want. All you can see from here is the other side of the hospital. It's not very attractive. The other side of the hall looks out onto the courtyard."

I never turned around to look at her. In my opinion, I had a beautiful view. I stood in fascination as I watched the men on the scaffold. There was a long period of silence before my dad said, "Christine, don't you think you ought to get in bed, Honey? You don't want to tire yourself out."

I looked into his eyes. In a tone of amazement I said, "Dad, look at the people! Look at the birds. And the sun. Dad, there's *life* out there!!" I placed my hand on the window in an effort to touch the life that was before me.

My smile was halted as I felt a twinge of pain in my heart. It was the recognition of reality. I reached out to the life that I cherished and was met by a cold hard barrier. That barrier was so much of a metaphor for who I really was. I could never bring the beauty of the world *inside* myself. It was always out there...I saw it...but could never *feel* it or live it. The birds, the sunshine, all the beauty of the world was someone else's happiness; not mine. In reality, my life was much like that glass window.

I was living behind a glass window. I could see everyone and everything. I could choose who would come into my life and who would stay out. I would watch and play like I was part of their world, but in reality. . . I was alone.

I got in bed and pulled up the covers. I laid there for hours thinking about the analogy of the glass window. It amazed me how I could have a drastic change of feelings and my dad would never notice. As long as I was "good" and exhibited the behavior that he viewed as "acceptable", everything was fine.

I watched him from inside my own glass window. I had not said a word in hours. He had not noticed that I was no longer smiling. I wasn't talking about the life I loved so much. When I stopped talking. . . he started doing. He made everything "perfect" in my room. He took the extra items that weren't functional to the car. He was taking my balloon bouquets, cards and posters home. He unpacked my suitcase and hung each item up in my closet. He filled my pitcher with water and straightened my towels. When he finished completing his tasks, he went to the lobby and bought a paper to read. He had been sitting in the chair by my bed since he returned.

I watched my dad and thought about how much I idolized him throughout my life. I was so emeshed in my father. I spent my life trying to please my dad. No matter what I did. . . it was never good enough. Although I could never win his approval, he had always been there for me. I was deep in thought when I was interrupted by Dad closing his newspaper. He said, "Well, its getting kind of late. I think I'll get me something to eat and then go on home. Do you need anything, Sweet-heart?"

I wanted to laugh. I thought, "Do I need anything? Yeah, I need something. I need *YOU* and I need you to quit being so demanding." I wanted to take everything he had neatly arranged in my closet and throw it on the floor. I felt like screaming, "I'm sick of this! I hate being perfect. I'm sick of trying to please you. I'm sick of living in a morgue when there is life out there. I want to live, damn it! I'm sick of everything that I do - not being good enough for you." But I couldn't do it.

My love for my father was the deepest affection I held for anyone or anything. I wanted his approval and his acceptance more than I wanted to live. But we always went through the motions. We say a lot of "I love you's" and show affection, but feelings are something that are not easily discussed in my family. My feelings lived in the morgue with me behind my glass window. All Dad saw was the smile. And the constant "I love you, Daddy's". On the inside I was dying. No matter what I attempted I could *never* measure up to his expectations.

The more emotions I showed, the more he withdrew. The more I tried to tell him how I *really* felt, the more he interpreted those feelings as anger and hatred towards *him*. He said, "if that's the way you feel, then maybe it would be best if I just got out of your life." I was angry at Dad for making me feel guilty. He had done so much for me. He didn't have to straighten up my new room. He was trying to make things nice for me. As I looked at him, I could see the hurt in his eyes due to my illness. And I was angry at him for hurting. Joe took the bulk of the emotional pain when I was sick the first time. He couldn't handle it and he left me. Then Dad took his place. He never left my side. I could see the pain in his face and it broke my heart. But he was on the other side of my glass window, too. He was doing what he thought was best, but he had no idea what I was feeling. And I couldn't tell him. Whenever I attempted, I became emotional. And like Joe . . . Dad despised that more than anything.

I remember one day at Dallas Community Hospital. It was before my transplant. I was given a drug that caused tremors much like convulsions. For the first time, he saw what goes on when "no one is allowed to come in." When I began trembling that day, Dad tried desperately to help me. He covered me with blankets. He tried to feed me ice chips. He poured water for me. He put a wet wash cloth on my forehead. He stroked my forehead. As the tremors intensified, Dad didn't know what to do. He tried everything to get his "little girl" to stop hurting on the outside. But I wanted him to make me stop hurting on the inside. I wanted him to show true unconditional love. I wanted him to really *listen to me and to* **approve of me.**

And I couldn't open my mouth to say a word to him. I just laid there and cried. I was so afraid I was going to lose him. I was afraid something was going to happen to him; that he couldn't handle my illness either and he would leave me.

I heard my doctor in the hallway. My tremors had calmed down. I asked Dad if he would go to the snacks-hop and buy me a candy-bar. It was a long walk to the snack shop. When he left my room, I went to the door and yelled to the nurse's station. I was supposed to be in isolation but I didn't care. "Will you ask Douglas to come in here real quick?" I yelled. "I'm okay, I just need to talk to him before Dad comes back."

I rolled my IV poles back to the bed and laid down. I was lying upside down when my doctor arrived. I had put my head on the pillow at the foot of the bed. He walked in and gave me a strange look. He turned his head sideways and said, "Isn't that suppose to go at the other end?"

I smiled and said, "Will you talk to Dad and tell him I'm okay? I think Dad thinks when I get sick, I'm getting worse." My voice cracked and I got tears in my eyes. "Douglas, he looked so helpless. You know Joe did the same thing. And I just. . ."

Dr. Douglas smiled at me and said, "I'll talk to him. You just keep getting sick." No matter how bad things were, he always made me laugh. Dr. Douglas talked to Dad without letting him know that I requested him to do so. Dad felt better and I felt better.

But it was only for the moment. I was still living behind my glass window. I had only postponed the pain. So many things were flashing through my mind when my dad's voice brought me back to the present reality.

"Do you want me to get you anything before I go?" he asked once again.

I just looked at him. I loved my dad immensely. I glanced at the window that so exemplified my life. It had gotten dark and I could not see outside. I looked at Dad and smiled.

"No. That's okay. I'm fine. I love you, Dad"

"I love you, too, Honey. I'll see you tomorrow morning," he said. He leaned over and gave me a kiss on the forehead.

I sighed as I looked out the window. "God, you've got to help me. I don't want to live in here anymore. But I don't know how to get to the other side."

I snuggled deep in my new bed. I turned on the television and thought, "Oh well, I'll think about it tomorrow."

The nurse came in and gave me my "sleeper" through an IV injection. I smiled as I felt the drug run through my veins and into my lungs. All the tension melted away. I continued to take deep breaths until I fell asleep.

God Bless you.
I hope you feel
better and have
a good rest to help
you get well.

Love,

MØ+T

PLEASE FIGHT FOR US. .
WE CANNOT FIGHT FOR OURSELVES"

# CHAPTER FIVE

## *Recovery of a Lifetime*

Dr. Mitchell arrived early the next morning and told me I needed a liver biopsy to find out if I definately had GVH. God, I hated that word! My body had been biopsied" so many times. I was surprised that a cure for cancer had not been discovered from my cells alone.

I got tears in my eyes after he left. I don't know why I had become so frightened of Graft vs. Host disease. Everyone who had a transplant had GVH to some degree. It comes and it goes. It's controlled by medications. The trick is to find the right combination of medications for the individual patient. Somewhere in my belief system, however, I thought GVH meant death. I found myself praying for hepatitis. Mom and Dad arrived soon after Dr. Mitchell left my room. I told them about the biopsy.

"Well good," Dad said. "When are they going to do it?"

I started to cry. "I don't know. I'm just so tired of all this. Am I going to die?"

My mother jumped up and started toward my bed. "So help me, God, Christine, if you say that one more time, I'm going to slap you right across the face. You're going to wish you had died!" she screamed. I started laughing.

She said, "I mean it. Now, you sit up in that bed, look out that window and read those cards that you got." That was my mother. She was the same mother she had always been. In other words she was saying, "You put that smile back on your face, you keep those feelings inside and you don't show *anybody* that you are afraid or hurt. . . or you are going to be punished."

As I watched her "display of affection", I became tickled. I could not stop laughing. "What are you going to do to me, Mom. . . kill me? I'm already dying," I said. She was laughing by this time also. It was as if something deep within me broke loose that day. The laughter came from a place deep within. I found a place inside of me with which I had never been. I think it is called "the other side." I knew that there was nothing my mother could do to hurt me.

I felt like I woke from the dead that day. The entire day was spent talking about the bone marrow transplant unit. I had been in the unit two days earlier, but I couldn't remember being there. I remembered bits and pieces. The entire experience was like a dark hole. It was that day my parents told me about seeing the birds in my bathtub, about George Washington being president of the United States and some other things that I had done. We laughed and we cried.

A nurse who had been off-duty entered my room. She said, "I just had to meet you. I was parking my car to come to work and I saw the 18-wheeler pull up out back and unload all your meds. I've just never seen a person take so many pills at once. Can I watch?" I looked at the tray. There were four cups with pills in them. We counted them. At the start of my recovery I was taking 54 pills a day.

The biopsy was scheduled for the following day. I don't remember a lot about the biopsy or the days surrounding it. I do remember being put on a pain medication. I remember it frightened me because I was so excited about having a narcotic prescribed. I never took drugs. I had no desire to do so. I would much rather "take care of the druggies." That was my drug of choice. With the amount of pain in my life at the time of the brain hemorrhage, it provided the perfect setting for chemical dependency. It started with the dilaudid.

Dilaudid produced the most incredible sensation that I have ever experienced. But I also knew it was a lie. Alcohol and drugs was the source of the pain in my life. I saw what it did to Joe. I worked in the field of Human Resources. I saw how it destroyed so many precious lives. Dilaudid was an excellent teacher. I learned how to manipulate various drugs to achieve the effect for which I was striving. But this time was going to be different. Instead of using the drug to anesthetize the pain, I used it to face the pain. When the narcotic was administered through the IV, I waited a few minutes for it to completely get into my system. I could feel it enter my vein. That was always my clue to start breathing deeply.

Although I was tempted to "get my fix", I did not do it. Instead, I visualized the pain medication traveling to the liver and the muscles surrounding it. As the pain dissipated, I pulled myself up in bed. I did sit ups to exercise that area. I used the numbness to get my muscles in shape. I continued this process through the night. Within a couple of days I was fine. There was no pain in that area. I no longer needed the medication.

The biopsy was definitive. I had Graft vs. Host disease. Dr. Mitchell was wonderful. He said, "We know what we're dealing with. We'll just take care of it." He was right. Within a few days, it was under control.

Dr. Mitchell said, "I've been trying to find a reason to keep you here. But I just can't find a good reason. Your GVH is under control. You don't have any infections or fevers . . . unless you *want* to stay . . . I think it's time for you to go home.

Although I was still having trouble walking and was extremely weak, I jumped out of bed. When he told me that I could go home . . . I didn't want to see that bed. I didn't want to touch it. It represented death to me. I wanted to live.

Dr. Mitchell said, "Now understand that most everyone has to come back to the hospital at some time. Most people will start running a fever or get an infection. You'll probably have to be admitted a couple of times. It's normal. But I think you are at the point that we can treat you as an outpatient."

I looked at him straight in the eye. I said, "I'm not coming back! Once I get out that door, I am **not** coming back. We can have lunch, but I am **not** coming back." He smiled as though he was cheering on my determination.

"There is one thing though," I said. "Can I borrow your britches? Nothing I brought to the hospital fits." I had gained 40 pounds from the steroids. I could feel my skin stretching to its limits.

I was released from the hospital on May 29, 1990. Leaving the hospital was a terrifying experience after being in a protective environment for such an extended period of time. I was overcome with emotion as I felt the warmth of the afternoon sun on my face. Although I had a mask that covered everything except my eyes, I could smell the freshness of the spring day.

There was so much activity. It was almost too much to take in at one time. People were walking at such a fast pace. I jumped as I heard the brakes of a car squeak. The birds seemed to have amplifiers as they chirped on the telephone pole. All the instructions I was given were going through my mind: "Don't let your skin be exposed to the sun . . . wear long sleeves . . . you won't have an immune system for a year to a year and a half so you have to be careful. . . wear your masks and gloves. . . don't go outside." I tried to combat the fear that the thoughts were creating.

Then I started thinking about all my responsibilities. I had a business to run. I had bills to pay. My yard.

. . who was going to take care of it? And my God, I was still married!!! It was as if I had forgotten about that part of my life. Thinking about the other patients who had transplants petrified me. So many of them had died from complications. A lot of them went back to work too soon and got sick. I was so tired of death and pain. I was tired of being afraid. And I was afraid to "give up" because I was afraid that I would die. I still wasn't sure how I got through my "blue funk." I really wasn't even sure I had gotten through it. I just knew I wasn't dead yet.

The ride home was exhausting. My dad pulled the car in front of my house. I began to cry when I saw it. I loved my house so much. I looked around at my neighbors' homes. They had been so supportive when I was in the hospital. They had been cutting my grass since Joe moved out. I never asked them to do it. They just started doing it.

When I first arrived home, it took every bit of my energy to get up the stairs. When I arrived to the half-way mark, I would sit down and rest. It was all I could do to take a shower and get dressed in the morning. I attempted to put on my makeup. Each day presented a challenge in make up application. Due to my excessive shaking from medication, it was several weeks before I could put on mascara. Eyeliner didn't come for many months. I was gaining additional weight from Prednisone. My normal weight is 108. I was up to 158. Nothing I owned fit, so I wore "one-size-fit-all" outfits.

Most mornings it was all I could do to get dressed. I would be worn out afterwards. I forced myself to get out of bed and go downstairs daily. Most days, however, that was my primary task. I wouldn't have the energy to do anything except lie on the couch. But, at least, I wasn't in bed.

I made a point to never go out without my masks and gloves. I remained in virtual isolation for one year. No one was allowed to come in my house and I never went outside. If I did go outside - I would be covered from head to toe.

After a few months of recuperation, my mother would take me to my church every morning. The sanctuary is designed somewhat as a "theater-in-the-round." Since I couldn't work out and couldn't go outside and walk, I would walk laps around the sanctuary. I remember when I first started. I would have to hold on to the back of the pews. It was difficult to breathe with a mask on. I did not have the stamina to walk very far. I made it half-way around the sanctuary and would have to go home. I would be on the couch the rest of the day. Soon I found my endurance building up. It was not long before I was walking six laps a day. I continued to do that until flu season started. The fear of becoming sick became too great.

It was in July of that year that I received a letter from my employer. The letter stated I had been placed on disability retirement. I had lost my primary job. I decided to put myself to work, working for myself. Dad built shelves in the closet of my office and bought a computer for me. My aunt purchased a laser printer. Each day was spent on my sofa sorting files. I bought a software package that forecasted the next year's budget. I began planning for my financial future and the future of my company. I was fortunate that I had money from my business to live on. Each day I would get dressed as if I was going to work. I didn't put on a suit, but I did wear a skirt and blouse. I applied my make-up and put on my wig and tried to work as long as I could without wearing myself out.

As a little girl, I use to play "office." I never wanted to play "school" like most of my friends did. Dad would buy me various business forms and sales receipt books. I would pretend that I was a sales clerk. My friends would buy my toys and I would give them a receipt. At times during my recovery, I felt like that same little girl playing "office." But playing "office" was the best medicine I had. I continued living.

Joe had still not made any attempt to put closure on our marriage. I knew that it would be months before I was healthy enough to go to court to finalize the annulment. It was four months later when I was finally able to go to court. I wore my sterile masks and gloves. I was out of breath by the time we arrived at the courthouse, even though it was only half-a-block away from my attorney's office. It was on September 4, 1990 that the judge in the 25th District Court awarded me an annulment. After my attorney presented my case, the judge said, "Honey, you can have anything you want and you need to remember that. You deserve it. Take care of yourself."

As I approached the one year mark anniversary of my transplant, I began to experience debilitating anxiety. I had been in virtual isolation for twelve months. My contact with the human race consisted of my family and the medical staff during my monthly visits to the hospital. When I did go out, it was with sterile masks and gloves.

I tried to dismiss my fears by staying busy with projects. I set unrealistic goals for myself and began working from early dawn until dusk. I was still "playing office" since I had not returned to work. I found myself on a merry-go-round of tasks and activities that I could not get off. Each day the ride got faster and I became more frightened

Every morning I looked for the return of my leukemia. I stood in front of the mirror and searched my body for bruises. When I brushed my teeth, I would apply intense pressure to reassure myself that they would not bleed.

The same thoughts terrorized my mind daily. "My God, what if I fumble? What if someone tackles me? I have come so far." I had an immobilizing fear that if I quit fighting or if I "let go"- that I was going to die. After several weeks of this normal, but very unrealistic fear, I went for counseling. I told the therapist: "For three years, crisis has become my lifestyle. I don't know how to live a normal life anymore."

With my therapist's encouragement, I entered the codependency addiction recovery program at a local psychiatric hospital. Through a series of seminars, group activities and self exploration, I quickly learned that my immobilization was real. I was "stuck" from going on with my life because I was "stuck" in the past. I had overcome numerous obstacles. My freedom was in my own hands. It was directly linked to facing the pain and completing the grief process.

I decided to leave my glass window at home. I never went anywhere without my wig. My hair had started to grow back, but it was extremely short. I felt unattractive. I knew throughout my life I used my looks to manipulate and control people. It was my largest defense mechanism and my "safest" protection. During many summers, I lived at the beach. My hair was bleached blonde from the sun. I always had the darkest tan on the beach. Wherever I went, I knew I could turn heads. After a number of years that, too, became empty.

As we arrived at the hospital, I experienced extreme anxiety. I told myself, "Christine, you are check-ing yourself into the hospital. You are in the field of Human Resources. You have developed and managed employee assistance programs. You know what goes on here. There is nothing to be afraid of. On a cognitive level, I knew that was true. My emotional side did not understand. I felt like the same little girl that was going to be given away if she didn't behave.

Mom and Dad helped carry my luggage to the lobby. The program was an intense two-week program. I was told to bring few personal possessions. Washing machines and dryers were on each unit. And I would have time to wash for a change of clothes. I still managed to have three suitcases filled with clothes, makeup, blowdryer and other "essential" elements of my life. We waited in the lobby. I signed my name on the registration form. The receptionist told me, "Someone will be down in a few minutes to check you in." I noticed no one could get through the doors to the lobby unless they had the receptionist release the lock. My anxiety level increased.

"My God, I'm going to be locked in here," I thought.

I looked at my parents for their reaction. They both looked as though they were waiting for their reserved table in a restaurant. My dad was dressed in a suit. My mother had on a bright red dress. She had matching purse, earrings and shoes. Both of them had the same expression on their face. It was the same look I saw the night of the Christmas Eve service the year before.

A schedule of events was lying on the coffee table next to the couch where my dad was sitting. He had been looking at a magazine. He glanced down at the schedule and said, "I see where they have a nutrition class here, Christine. You need to make sure that you attend that!" Both of my parents were totally oblivious to why I was there.

"They also have a family group. Will you be coming to that, Dad?" I inquired.

Mom spoke for him, as she did on so many occasions. "We have to go to Kansas, Christine." I gritted my teeth to keep from screaming at her. We had made so much progress in our relationship, but now we seemed to be going back to square one. I realized the only person that I could change was myself. My parents decided to go to Kansas immediately upon my sharing with them about my decision to go to a "psychiatric" hospital. She had told her friends, "Christine has checked herself into a hospital that has 'psychology programs' to learn coping skills and stress management." She had listened to my counseling "lingo" for so long; she could now repeat it verbatim.

"Christine Michael?" The person standing at the door was calling my name. I looked up. It was a blonde woman dressed in normal street clothes. I laughed to myself. I had toured hundreds of treatment centers in the past. When it was my turn to be admitted to one, however, I still expected a nurse with a white uniform, white hat, white hose and shoes. She should have a syringe in one hand and a straight jacket in the other.

"I'm Christine Michael," I said. I stood up and started to walk toward her.

"Can we go with her?" my mother asked.

We walked down the long corridor. It was full of bright canvas art and beautiful pictures of mountain scenery. We arrived at the nurse's station where I was to leave all my possessions. The person escorting us through the hospital looked at my parents. "She needs to go through assessment. You can wait for her in the family room."

My parents appeared to be in pain. They both had tears in their eyes. Neither of them understood why I was going to a psychiatric hospital. It was difficult for them to let go. They had taken care of me for months.

Each had given up their own lives when I became ill. In reality, I am not sure they ever had their own life. None of us had our own identity apart from the other.

"Why don't you'll go ahead and go?" I said.

The Intake Coordinator led me into a small room that had a desk with a soft light blue lamp sitting on it. There was a wing back chair beautifully decorated. That is where I sat. She opened the desk drawer and pulled out an abundance of paper work to fill out. She would complete the forms. I just had to come up with the answers.

"Now you came in here for depression?" she asked.

I was surprised by her statement. I said, "No. I didn't come in her for depression." I reached out to look at the file. I wanted to make sure she had the right folder.

"You *are* Christine Michael, right?" she asked.

"Yeah. But I didn't come in here for depression." I leaned back in my chair. "I may have come in here because I'm *not* depressed. That's more the problem," I said as I laughed aloud. I explained to the woman what I had been through in the last few years.

"The norm in my life has become crisis. I don't know how to live a normal life anymore," I said. "I started to become frightened a few months ago." I started to tell her about the "Celebrate Life" party I was planning, about the book I was writing, and how I wanted to be back at work soon. Whenever I get frightened, I start performing. And before I know it. . I am in another crisis."

She continued to conduct the intake interview. When it was completed she showed me to my room. I had requested a private room since my immune system had still not recovered. I could not be around a lot of other people. The normal requirement is that each patient have a roommate. Under the circumstances an exception was made for me. I was assigned a private room.

I turned around to pick up my luggage and it was gone. I had one suitcase. "Where is my overnight bag and tote bag?" I asked.

"Well, we keep those locked up," she said. "You can check your blow dryer and razor - those kind of things - out at the nurse's station. Everything else will be placed in a plastic bucket that will be locked in the galley."

I must have looked at the woman like I thought she came from the "nut house." I thought, "She's not really a nurse. She's a patient. This is crazy! I checked myself in here. Now they are taking everything away? And I didn't even wear my wig. Oh, God, what have I done?" I felt like I was standing naked in the middle of downtown 5:00 P.M. traffic.

I suddenly realized they had my medications. They were in my tote bag. "What about my medications?" I asked in a dubious tone of voice. "I'm still on medication for my transplant and I have to have those at various times of the day." I began to panic.

"You will have a physical with the doctor tomorrow. Just tell him what you are taking. You can then request it from the nurse's station," she said.

"But I have to have it tonight!" My voice was getting more defensive.

"I'm on duty tonight. I'll get it for you," she said. I was almost in tears.

I entered my room. I turned around with my "smiley face" and said, "Thank you. It was so nice meeting you. I'll see you later."

My room looked much like a college dorm room. It had twin beds, two small closets and a dresser. There was no television or radio. I took my suitcase to the closet and began to unpack the limited number of outfits I had brought with me. After hanging everything up in it's proper place, I instinctively glanced to look at my reflection in the mirror. There was no mirror. I could not see myself and that terrified me. I think it was at that moment I realized how empty my life really was. I didn't have a role to play. Without a role I did not know who I was. I desperately wanted to run away. But I made myself stay. I laid on my bed and cried for hours.

I glanced at my watch and realized that Group Orientation was only an hour-and-a-half away. I decided that I would be the "perfect" psych patient and read my material. As I reached over to grab the packet of information that was given to me upon admission, I remembered something I had brought to the hospital with me. It was in my purse. I pulled it out and began to read. It was titled "Autobiography in Five Short Chapters." It read:

I

*I Walk Down the Street*
*There is a manhole in the sidewalk*
*I fall in*
*It isn't my fault*
*It takes forever to find a way out.*

## II

*I walk down the Street*
*There is a manhole in the sidewalk*
*I fall in again*
*It isn't my fault.  It still takes a long time to get out*

## III

*I Walk down the Street*
*There is a manhole in the sidewalk*
*I still fall in.  My eyes are open.*
*It is my fault.*
*I find a way to get out.*

## IV

*I walk down the Street*
*There is a manhole in the sidewalk*
*I walk around it*

## V

*I take another Street.*

Ironically, the hospital I was in distributed the handout at a training session that I scheduled for supervisors of my company.  It was part of their training for the new employee assistance program.  The topic was "chemical dependency and other addictions: how to recognize it in your employees." I had started an employee resource center where employees could check out video tapes, books, audio tapes or files on about any subject imaginable.  I made a copy of the handout for my files.  When I first read the autobiography, I remember thinking, "That is the most ridiculous thing I have ever read in my life."  As I read it that night, it was apparent to me why I had checked into the hospital.

I had been walking down that same street all of my life. I was no longer falling in the manholes. I was exhausted from walking around them. At one time the manhole represented everything I wanted: it was my security and it was my identity. But now - all it represented was pain. I wanted to take another street, but I just did not know how. I didn't know what that street looked like; much less how to get there. But I was determined to find out. No matter what it took, I was going on. I pulled myself up from the bed as I heard someone knock on my door. Without waiting for my response, they entered. It was the nurse that conducted my intake interview. She had someone with her. At first I thought the person was crying.

"Christine, this is your roommate," she said as she introduced the woman to me.

I said, "There must be a misunderstanding. I have a private room."

"All patients have roommates," she replied.

My desire to please was overtaken by my desire to live. I looked at the woman who was supposed to be my roommate. Her eyes were red and swollen. She coughed and covered her nose as she sneezed. She had a terrible cold.

I looked back at the nurse. I said, "I understand that. But this was cleared with Administration before I was ever admitted. I had a bone marrow transplant and I have to be real careful since I don't have an immune system."

The nurse explained to me there were no other rooms available. "The only other room is on the locked psychiatric unit. I can't do that to her."

I wanted to say, "Do it to me. I'll go on the locked unit. I've been locked up for a lot longer than two weeks. Two weeks is nothing."

The woman that was assigned to be my roommate began to cry. She felt guilty because they had given her to me as a roommate. Then I felt guilty for making her cry and for saying what I had said.

As always I said, "That's okay. I brought my masks and stuff so it's okay. I'll leave you'll alone. I'm going to go get a drink of water." I walked out of the room and I began to cry. I was so afraid I was going to die. I had come so far. Of all people they could put me with. . . I had to get a roommate that had walking pneumonia. I looked around and there was **no where** to go. Patients were not allowed to leave the unit without a staff escort, outside was off limits and we weren't allowed to use the phone. I knew I had a choice. I could "bolt" and run or I could stick it out. I was too frightened to do either one. I stood against the wall on the unit, threw my head back and said with a deep sigh, "God, you've got to help me find another street!"

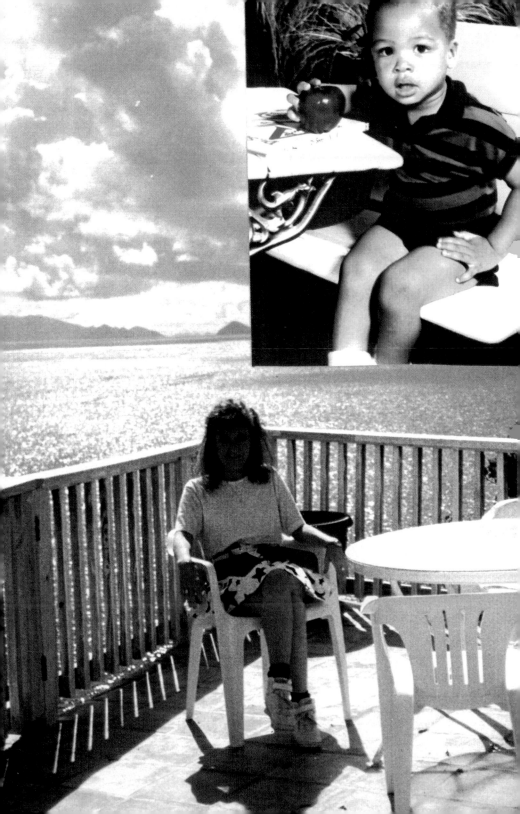

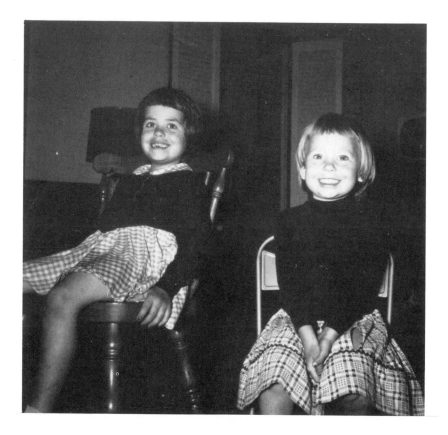

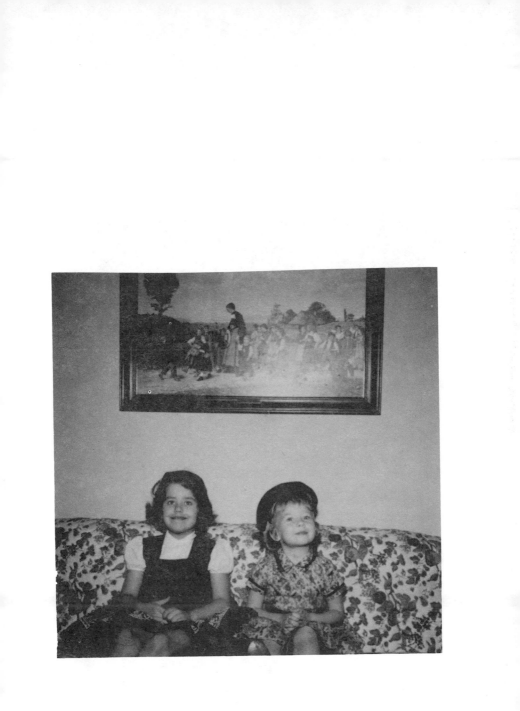

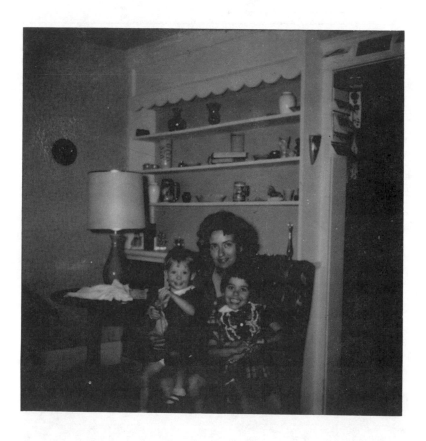

# CHAPTER SIX

## *Releasing the Pain*

It was 6:30 A.M. when someone knocked on my door. "Wake-up," he yelled. We had been told in orientation that we were expected to have our beds made each morning. I couldn't remember the last time I made my bed. The majority of time in the last year had been spent in the bed. By 7:00 A.M. we were to meet in the lounge. We were going to the gym for fitness time. After exercising we were given 30 minutes to get ready before we were required to be at breakfast. I hate breakfast. I laid in my bed and thought, "I can't believe I have done this to myself."

The idea of having to get dressed to go to the nurse's station and request my medication infuriated me. I was experiencing more anxiety than I could handle. I kept thinking, "I gave them the prescriptions. I'm the one that told **them** what I was taking. Now I have to go ask for it?" I decided to take a shower first. I entered the bathroom. Then I realized they had my soap, my shampoo, my razor. . . I got back in bed and pulled the covers over my head. I thought, "Maybe I can hide and they won't realize I'm missing."

It seemed as though just a few moments had passed when I heard. . . "Breakfast." Some man was yelling through the hallway. I pulled the covers down from over my face and looked at my roommate. Her nose was red and she was crying. I closed my eyes and thought, "God, is there not **anywhere** that I can go and be happy?"

I went to the cafeteria and sat with some people in my group. There was a couple of people that had been released from the "locked side." I decided they had graduated from the group who was insane to the group that was going insane. The winner of the "Mrs. America" contest was in my group. She and I got along well. We talked about how to apply makeup. A couple of people had been given and ultimatum by their spouses. That is why they were there. A man who I had not met came over to the table. He sat with us. He thought he was Adolph Hitler. By lunchtime, he was Napoleon and that evening - he became Alexander the Great. He and I became good friends. He had so many different personalities; it was easy for me to keep pace. I could play whatever role he needed. That's what I had done all my life.

The first day was exhausting. From 6:30 A.M. to 9:30 P.M. we were mandated to eat, exercise and go to workshops. We had 30 minutes to reflect on the day. Lights were to be out at 10:00 P.M. Each of us was pulled aside during the day to be examined by a medical doctor, a psychiatrist and to have our blood pressure and temperature taken. Each workshop had homework to be completed. We were required to keep a journal. My therapist had given me an autobiography questionnaire to complete. It dealt with my family of origin. It had the questions written down. I just had to come up with the answers. Before entering the hospital, I "conveniently" lost the questionnaire several times. My therapist was never surprised when I misplaced it. She would just smile and say, "You have a lot of practice, Christine, at avoiding things you don't want to face. You've had to for survival. It doesn't surprise me that you lost it."

I adored my therapist. Having a degree in Counseling, I knew all the theories. I knew the systems of counseling. The thing that I loved about this hospital and treatment center is that the counselors develop a treatment and recovery program for the clients from the first day of therapy. There is not much time spent on talking and reflecting. The therapists guide each person through a journey based on his particular needs and wants. Each patient gets a teddy bear when they arrive.

Since my treatment began before hospitalization I was already aware of the teddy bears. After seeing that I was "stuck" in a process my therapist asked me, "Christine, do you have any teddy bears?"

"Do I have teddy bears?  My house is full of them." I told her that I had delivered a stillborn baby boy and the nursery was decorated in teddy bears.

"Is there one that you are particularly close to? One that you have a fondness for?" she asked.  I thought about my "little leukemic bear" that I loved dearly; a part of my Christmas celebration. . .he wore a sterile mask, sterile gloves and a big red bow-tie. I said, "There's definitely a bear that I feel attached to." I did not tell her which one or why I felt particularly fond of the bear.

She said, "I want you to do something. This may be a little embarrassing.  You don't have to do it when there is a crowd around.  I want you to take the bear to the mall.  You need to carry that bear as if it was your little girl.  Now I want you to buy an outfit for that little girl, but buy her what *she* wants to wear. And you need to take care of her. Bring her back next week.  And Christine. . . find your autobiography."

In an effort to complete my homework assignment the following day, I picked up the bear and headed toward the door. The apprehension increased.  My heart was beating fast Glancing toward the kitchen I thought, "I'll put him in a paper bag. I don't have to actually carry him into the mall." I knew I couldn't do that either. I had a degree in Counseling. I wasn't stupid. I knew that this experience had more to it than taking a stuffed animal to a store and buying it something to wear. That "little leukemic bear" was so familiar to me because it was the real me. It was the Christine who loved Christmas. And who loved to play . . and who lived behind a glass window.

A meeting had been scheduled for the following day with the fund-raising committee that I was chairing. I decided I would go to a mall on the other side of town before the meeting. I rationalized the solution to my impasse by saying, "You don't have to do it all in one day, Christine. You know what's going on. You can deal with it." The next morning I overslept. I never made it to the mall. I tried one other time, but I broke out in an excessive rash. That prompted me to begin searching my body for bruises. The following week I returned to my therapist's office with a naked teddy bear.

On an intellectual level I knew what was going on with me. Yet emotionally - I was immobilized from doing anything about it. Once again. . . my therapist was not surprised. "Christine, let's just put your little girl in the chair. She's feeling real vulnerable and scared right now. You and I will talk," she said. I reached over and put "my inner child" in the chair across from me. I was sitting in the chair next to my therapist's desk so I could turn my head and look at her. I did not have to look at the bear.

We talked about my autobiography. I had managed to bring it with me that time. I even had a large part of it filled out. I had stopped when I got to the portion where I had to write about my dad. We talked about expectations and about approval. We discussed the issue of shame.

Somewhere during the conversation my therapist maneuvered the focus back on to the child that lived inside of me; the child that was never allowed to express her feelings. "Christine, look at that little girl sitting in the chair. What does she want you to know? What is it that she wants to tell you?" she asked.

I looked over at that precious child and for the first time. . . I saw myself. I saw that little 3-year-old that was so happy. All she wanted was to love and be loved, to laugh and to play.  She loved singing and dancing and she loved life.

I looked at her and my heart sank.  Not only did I see that adorable child with golden blonde hair, big blue eyes and a smile that never quit, but I also saw what I had done to her all her life.  I saw the tear-stained eye and the mask that disguised her entire being.

I turned my head and looked at my therapist. Tears were streaming down my face.  "I can't look at her," I said as I covered my face.

My counselor didn't reply.  She sat and waited until I was ready to uncover my face and invite her in. I took my hand down from my face, looked up at the ceiling and sighed.  I breathed deeply, bit my lip and looked at my therapist.  She had not moved.  She never changed her expression.  I felt the most incredible love coming from her. But more importantly - I felt accepted. She had not reached out toward me when I was strug-gling.  She didn't have to.  She had never moved.  It was much the same type of love I received from God the night I sat on my staircase and cried.

I looked over at the child that had been buried for so many years. Those big blue eyes melted my heart. "My God, I'm killing her," I said.  "She's suffocating behind that mask.  She is dying."

"What does she want to tell you, Christine?"

I heard that small voice within me my heart.  "I love you," it said.

"That she loves me," I replied.  I made myself look her in the eye.  I looked at the locket I had made her.  It was hanging around her neck.  It had my picture in it.  In the photograph I was smiling much like she would. But I was an imposter. I looked at her tear stained eye.

I continued. "And that she wants to live. She's tired of living behind that mask." For the first time I was daring to look within my own heart. I continued to listen for that voice that was crying out in desperation. ". . And she wants to be like me," I said. My entire body felt pain as I made that comment.

I tried to listen more closely. "No!! She doesn't want to be like me. She wants **me** to be like her." I looked to my therapist for confirmation. She smiled and raised her eyebrows. I knew that I had found the beginning of my truth. I had started on my journey. I was no longer inside looking out. The glass had been broken.

"Can you do that? Can you give her that?" she asked.

I looked at the precious child and looked at the woman that had just introduced me to myself. The child was filled with love - It was as if she was saying, "Here I am. Come get me. I love you. I want to live with you."

The love and forgiveness that inner child was offering was overpowering. I did not know how to give it back. The little girl that lived inside of me was so full of life and love and laughter. She didn't want anything in return. She just wanted to love.

I closed my eyes and tried to determine a way I could take her with me. It saddened me greatly when I realized she would have to stay. I didn't know how to give her what she needed. I returned to the reality of my pain. My therapist was waiting for my reply.

"I don't know how," I said. "I have absolutely **no** idea how to take care of her. I know I don't want to go back to where I was. The pain is too great. But I don't know how to get to get to the other side."

It was as if that glass window had been broken. There was nothing preventing me from breaking free; yet I was immobilized. I didn't know how to get from the inside to the outside. That was my reality. It had become my life. It was at that point that my therapist encouraged me to check into the hospital. I was stuck. I needed to learn how to take care of myself.

The third day at the hospital I was scheduled to have a private session with my therapist. I could not wait. The sessions I had attended in the hospital were so intense. Working through the pain was almost debilitating at times. I was running a low grade fever and my blood pressure was elevated. My therapist led one of our workshops and told me she would meet with me after lunch. She was waiting for me when I entered the room. I was surprised to find three white boards in the room. She had a planned agenda.

"Christine, I want you to list for me all the things you have been through in the last few years. We're going to take this in bite-size-chunks." I must have looked bewildered.

"Just start listing. When did it all start?" she asked.

"Well, I guess it started when my grandfather died." Then I told her the whole story about that event. Then I would go to the next item. Somewhere along the lower half of the second board I listed "delivered stillborn baby boy." I continued and began to write on the third board.

"Wait a minute," she said. "That's enough for now. I want to ask you something. What would you say about a person that had been through all of this stuff? That's *a lot* of pain."

As I looked at the boards filled with tragedy I commented, "I would wonder how she got through it."

"Exactly," she said. "Christine, let's go back up here. What does this say?"

"Delivered still born baby boy." It was always difficult for me to say those words unless I said it quickly and in passing.

"Had you'll named the baby?" she asked.

"Well. . . yeah. We were going to name it Christopher Michael if it was a boy," I said.

"Write that up there next to that," she said. She then told me to continue my list. Upon nearing comple- tion - I ran out of board space. She said, "That's okay. Let's go back to this one. Christine, what does this say?"

"Delivered still born baby boy Christo. . . " My words were halted by the lump in my throat. The pain was so great that it impeded my vocal chords. My eyes began to fill with tears.

"Christine, what does that say?" she repeated. My lips quivered as I tried to speak. Tears were stream- ing down my face.

"Delivered still born baby boy. . . " I hesitated while I struggled to get the last part of my sentence out. "Christ. . . opher. . . Michael"

"Say it again, Christine."

"Delivered still born baby boy - Christopher Michael," I said as I burst into tears. I sat in my chair and covered my face with my hands.

"I wanted my baby!" I screamed. My heart was shattered as I verbalized his name for the first time.

"You wanted who, Christine?"

"I wanted Christopher Michael!" I wailed as I fell to the floor in agony. "I **still** want Christopher Michael!" Christopher Michael. . . Oh God, I want him. I love him. I miss him." I let out a blood curdling scream.

"That's right," she said. "Christine, say it one more time. You want who?"

I couldn't breathe I was sobbing so heavily. "I want Christopher Michael. I still want Christopher Michael." My body collapsed on the floor.

"Christine, you have **never** grieved over any of this stuff. You've done some. But when it comes to Christopher Michael - you have not even begun the grief process."

"Who had time to grieve?" I asked as I began to pull myself up from the floor. "I couldn't stand the pain. Just one of those things was enough to kill me," I said.

"I want you to spend the entire weekend grieving, Christine. I don't want you to wear any makeup or jewelry. Just spend the weekend grieving. Go to your sessions, but **grieve**, Christine."

"Okay," I said as I looked at a 3-year-crisis that I truly *did* wonder how I got through. I was looking at each event when I realized that I did not know how to grieve.

I looked at my therapist. "I don't know how to do that," I said.

"I know you don't. Christine, just **be**. Make a list of the events you have been through, attach the feeling you had with each and bring it into the present. Grieve, Christine, You have got to grieve!" she said.

As I left the session with my therapist, I wanted to play. I did not want to deal with the pain. I thought, "Well, I know what the problem is. I'll just take care of it later. My mind saw that precious little 3-year-old that loved to play. That's what I wanted to do. . . laugh and play. That's who I was deep down. I knew that was true. "Why do I have to grieve now? I've already been through so much pain. I don't want to go through it again," I thought.

I spent a day-and-a-half trying to grieve. I wore no makeup or jewelry. I went to the cafeteria and sat alone. I didn't smile and I didn't play "Suzy Sunshine." But I still felt like I was playing a role. I didn't really feel the pain. It was buried deep within me. All I was doing was putting on the "face of grief." I didn't have a clue what I was doing. My assignment was to grieve and *I **didn't know how!*** My frustration level was increasing.

I had gotten in touch with that little girl inside of me. She wanted to live. I wanted to live! After much avoidance, I decided I would try what my counselor had suggested. I began to list the crisis that had occurred in the past few years. I closed my eyes to help focus on when it all began. I thought about my childhood. That wasn't it. It may have started there, but I knew my parents did the best they could. I thought about David, an old boyfriend. He had hurt me deeply.

"I guess I better start there," I thought.

I began to write. "I ran into David after 10 months of being apart. I had told him to never call me again. I was doing well and had gone on with my life. We got together to talk. He told me he thought we should be together and wanted to marry me. I had been through eight years of a roller-coaster ride with David. When he was ready for a commitment, I wasn't. Then when I became ready he would say, "I just don't feel that way." I finally opened up my heart again. I told David I would give it a try and start seeing him. I let down my guard. I told him that I would marry him. Within three weeks he was back out the door. Date: 5/87 Feeling: I was traumatized."

Then I remembered my grandfather had died a few months earlier. . . . "I was on my way to see him that weekend. It was his birthday. He had a stroke and died before I arrived. Date: 2/87 Feeling: sadness. I went to the funeral home to spend some time with him - just by myself. It was the first time I ever touched anyone that was dead. I gave him a kiss on the cheek when I was standing next to the casket. I stroked his face. I loved him more than anyone in this world. He was the **only** person in my life I ever felt truly loved me. He always "showed me off" to his friends. He called me his "little chocolate kid." We use to go for long walks when I was little. I was Pa-Pa's shadow. Wherever he went - I went. We walked to the coffee shop every morning when I stayed with him. I'd get chocolate ice cream and he would get a cup of coffee. He's put ice in his coffee. I miss him terribly."

This process continued for hours. I was in my room writing as quickly as I could. I would cry some and then re-read what I had written. It was close to 10:00 P.M. My roommate was trying to sleep.

The hospital had a room that was called a "quiet room." It was soundproof so you could scream. It was also padded in order that you could "appropriately" display your feelings. I hate that word. . . appropriately. I decided I would go to the "quiet room" so that I could scream and cry. That would be the "appropriate" way to grieve.

I spent four hours in that room crying and writing. I remember thinking, "My God, they're never going to let me out of here. I'm not even up to 1989. Oh God. . . help me," I cried. I was nauseated from sobbing so intensely. And I had this unquenchable desire to play miniature golf. I hated crying. It always made me sick to my stomach. I would cough and gag because I couldn't breathe. I said to myself, "No wonder I don 't grieve. This is the pits." I left the "quiet room."

One of my favorite therapist was playing "guard duty" on our wing. When I approached the desk she smiled and said, "Hi, Christine." I stopped to talk with her.

"Pam, will you help me?" I asked. "I'm sick of this crap. I have written 40 pages and I am not even up to 1989. I have cried so much I am about to throw up. I have an excruciating headache. I don't know what to do. It's like the pain is screaming to get out of my body, but it won't come out."

She looked down and giggled. "Oh, Christine. You are so funny. You're still trying to do it up here," she said as she pointed to her head. "Get it down here in the gut. You just need to feel it."

As she made that statement, I thought, "Who in the hell wants to feel it? It almost killed me when I went through it the first time."

"You know what you are doing? You are trying to grieve the "right" way. It's like you're writing down all of the events so then you can attach the "right" feeling to it and then bring it to the present. You just need to grieve. Keep it out of your head. You are still trying to process cognitively. She smiled as she tried to convey how difficult I was making my own life.

"Christine, why don't you just try writing a letter to the pain?" she suggested. Her suggestion "felt right". I didn't know how I was going to accomplish the task, but I did know somewhere in the process of writing that letter - I would find my answer. That night was the start of my recovery.

I went back to my room. I tried to be quiet as I opened the door. My roommate was sleeping. I turned on the light over my bed. According to the rules, lights were to be out four hours earlier. I took my "encyclopedia of crisis" and laid it on the nightstand. I thought about doing the polite thing by turning off the light so I would not disturb my roommate. That is what I would have always done in the past. That night was different. I refused to go through another day with the pain left inside of my heart. I knew I was on the right track. I refused to quit before I found my answer. I started to write when I heard a voice within my say, "Don't edit your words. Just get your feelings out." I began to write.

*For the sake of respecting the boundaries of others, the offensive language has been edited from this manuscript*

Dear Pain:

I hate your _____ guts! I despise what you've done in my life. I was so happy at one time. You took a child that was so precious, and so loving and giving. She was vulnerable and you almost killed her with your ___ _____ critical attitude. Even now - as she is starting to live again. . . you try to smother her and keep her inside. I want you dead. I want to kill you. You

are not worth one once of energy. You deserve
to die and burn in Hell forever. I speak everything bad on your ability to continue existing. I
hate you for killing Christopher Michael. I want
him so desperately. I miss him. I never even got
to see his face and it's all your _____ fault. I
hate you for taking Joe away from me. I loved
him with every ounce of my being.  I want to
take knives and stab you until you have no life
left inside of you. I want to you to hurt the way
that I hurt.  I hate you for robbing me of my 33
years of existence.   My parents made some
mistakes but they **did** love me. And you made
me feel like I wasn't good enough. Well____you,
damn it. I am good enough.  And my parents
are good enough. Well, you know what,_____
___ ____, I have parents who love me, I have a
God who loves me and I have an inner child who
loves me.  And I love her - And I am going to
take care of her. You're the one that doesn't
know how to take care of her; not me.  So you
can't come into my life anymore.

I will never cut off my feelings again. I will never
allow shame to enter my life.  I make mistakes.
I am human. But I learn from those mistakes. It's
not bad to hurt. And it's not bad to feel angry.
But it is **NOT** okay to keep that pain inside. You
will never be able to hold me down again
because I don't just want to kill you - I **DO** kill
you.

I have my little girl with me and I'm holding her
by the hand.  She trusts me now. And I trust me
because I know that it's not me that wants to
hurt her - it's you.  And you want to hurt me.
Well, you're not going to. Because I want to live.

I'm going to live! You _____ idiot. I see you
melting like the witch in the Wizard of Oz. (Ding

Dong the Witch is Dead). I choose to be healthy. I choose to be free. And I choose for you to no longer keep me down. I have informa tion and I now have skills. I will use my resourc es. I will no longer walk around those manholes.

By God-
I'm taking another street! ! ! ____ you. Go to Hell! I'm Free! You even had me trying to ____-____ grieve the "right way." ____ you, you power-less spineless creature. YOU'RE DEAD! ! ! ! ! !

As I completed the letter, an incredible peace came over me. The pain was gone. I looked around waiting for a bolt of lightening to strike my for my language. Instead I heard a voice within me say, "That a girl!"

I started to pray. I said, "God, why is that I just did something that ordinarily I would feel so guilty about and that is so contrary to what I believe I "should" do. And I feel closer to you now than I ever have before. I always thought "taking your name in vain" was equivalent to murder."

Once again, I heard a voice within me say "Christine, those are **words**. It's not the intent of your heart. You make your own interpretation. I have so much for you. I love you. I look at your heart. I **live** within your heart. You spend so much time searching for me. All you have to do is look within your own heart. It is there that you will find me. Why is it so hard for you to believe that I love you? I have told you, "I will never leave you nor forsake you."

I wasn't real sure who was speaking to me. I didn't know if was God, or my "higher power," the Holy Spirit, my inner child or if it was merely myself. What I did know is that the pain was gone and I had a peace that I had never experienced before. And for the first time. . . I knew I had a God who loved me just the way I  was.

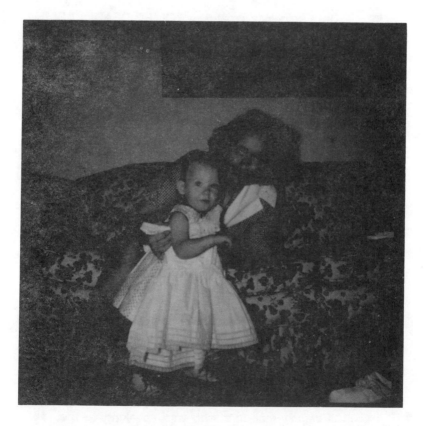

# CHAPTER SEVEN

## *The Most Beautiful View In the World*

I was released from the treatment center and was so excited about being alive. I had been so afraid that I was going to die when I entered the hospital. I had all the symptoms that my roommate had; a chronic cough, fever, tight chest, sore throat. . . but I didn't die. I got sick, but I didn't die. I took medicine like normal people. I got over it and I lived. Upon exiting the center, I created a follow-up plan to stay in recovery. I set goals in every area of my life: physical, spiritual, mental and emotional.

I made two major commitments before I entered the hospital. One was the first "Because I Care Tissue Typing Day," an event to increase world-wide awareness of the need for bone marrow donors. I was chairing the Life-Link auction. And I also planned a party for my birthday on April 5. It was a party for everyone to come together and celebrate life. It was promoted as a "thank you for your love and support" party.

The invitations to the party were filled with cartoon characters like Mickey Mouse and Donald Duck. The decorations were bright lime green, bright blue, yellow, red and bright pink. I ordered 400 helium balloons that had the words "Celebrate Life" printed on them.

A patient who had his transplant the week after mine also had his birthday the week after mine. I called him and told him I would love to include him in the celebration if he would like to be a part of it.

Friday, April 5, 1990 approximately 450 people came to my "Celebrate Life" party. I celebrated my thirty-third birthday.  But it was a day for everyone to come together and celebrate the precious life that God had given each of us. The highlight of the event was a hypnotist. He took my idea of a "mental" balloon ride into the heavens and turned it into something extraordinary.

The hypno-therapist had us close our eyes. He began to take us on a beautiful balloon ride journey..."As you begin to rise from this lovely meadow you feel an incredible peace and love. You feel secure and protected. You can smell the aroma of the grass below and the fragrance of the flowers. You can feel the warmth of the sunshine on your face. As you continue to rise you are safely resting in the guidance of this magical balloon. You feel loved and you feel safe. You feel accepted just the way you are. You can hear the birds singing. As you approach the soft clouds, you feel the gentle breeze of the morning air. You begin to feel comfort and love radiating from the clouds. You are drawn closer. As you continue to rise, you see a bright, beautiful light. Out of this light comes a mighty hand stretching out to meet you. It is the hand of God. In this hand...there is a dove. And the dove has something in it's mouth. It is a bag. The bag is for you. The dove flies to meet you on your journey. It lands on your shoulder and you see that it has something in the bag. The bag is full of gifts for you. It is filled with the innermost desires of your heart. It's full of love, peace...a healing for your illness, acceptance..whatever it is that you are in need of tonight. Picture yourself taking those gifts out of the bag. They are yours. Receive them for yourself. And there are some things in your life that are weighing you down and making your journey heavy. God wants to release you from those things. Whatever it is that is keeping you in pain; that's keeping you from moving on about your journey...your divorce, the death of a child or grandchild...the loss of a special relationship...the child in you that never received the love you deserved...whatever that little secret place in your heart is hiding...picture yourself putting those things into the bag. Tonight is the night to get rid of those things. You don't have to hurt anymore. As you put those things in the bag, you feel yourself becoming lighter. . ."

The therapist led us back to the meadow and then to the room in which we were sitting. He asked us to take the imaginary bag that we had encountered on our journey and tie it to the helium balloon attached to our chair. Each of us took a helium balloon. We went outside and simultaneously released them to God. It was a beautiful experience to see hundreds of balloons being released at the same time. It was a night to "let go" and to begin to celebrate life. That is why it was called a "Celebrate Life" party. Several television shows taped the event and newspapers were there to cover the story.

After the party, my "one-year-out" post-transplant check-up was approaching. I heard my "inner voice" tell me something. "Christine, why don't you get a mammogram while you are seeing the doctor?" the voice said. I had learned to listen to that inner voice, so I scheduled a mammogram. My mammogram turned out to be abnormal. It was carcinoma, but the lump was so small, it was easy to treat. The doctor said that due to early detection, I would never see the cancer again! That was a wonderful birthday present.

Just a few weeks later, however, I received the best birthday present that I could have ever had. Saturday, April 20 was the auction. It was a fundraiser for "tissue typing" bone marrow donors, a necessary step in the search for much needed donors. At the auction Dr. Douglas made a phone call to a man in Peebles, Scotland...a man named John Falla. He was a 40 year-old man who for no reason except to give to his fellow man... and because he knew that there was a 31 year old woman that was dying - decided to donate his marrow to save her life. When God made John and me, He made us so much alike that our bone marrow was identical; a 1:20,000 chance. A major newspaper reporter in our city wrote an article about the event. The reporter asked me what would be the first question that I was going to ask my donor.

Ever since my transplant, I have freckles all over my face. I never had them before. I questioned Dr. Mitchell for a year concerning the reasons for the development of my freckles. He never would give me a straight answer. I said "I bet you my donor has freckles." He assured me that had nothing to do with it. Everyone in the audience had a copy of the article. I was trying to keep the focus on marrow donation.

"John, what made you decide that you wanted to donate?" I asked. "Did you have someone in your family that had leukemia?"

"Well, over here, it's kind of like charity. You know. . . just giving to your fellow man," he said.

"John, that's such a sacrifice."

"Oh, no, Christine, it's no sacrifice. You had the hard part. I had the easy part."

"Did you find it painful?" I asked.

"Oh, gosh no," he said. "Let's see. It's kind of like maybe I played rugby or soccer too long. It was like pulling a muscle or something."

I had been so involved in the phone call I had almost forgotten there was anyone else in the room. I looked up. As I lifted my head, I saw three people on the front row in tears. It was then that I realized what had happened in my life. The man on the other end of the phone was literally the one man that could save my life. He had the unselfishness to give to a woman that he knew nothing about. He had not known anyone that had leukemia. He only knew there was a 31 year old woman that was dying. As I looked into the audience, I realized that although I was standing in Mesquite, Texas, I was talking to a man in Peebles, Scotland. I had his blood running through my body and his bone marrow manufacturing my blood cells. After the transplant, whenever I talked about my donor, my mind always saw a "bag of marrow" hanging on an IV pole. It now had a voice. It was a flesh and blood human being. And he had given me life.

I told him, "John, if it weren't for you I wouldn't be standing here. You are *literally* the one person who could save my life. I can't believe you did that; and never even knew anyone that had leukemia."

In a humble tone he said, "Oh no, Christine. You are alive. That is the important thing." I was overcome with emotion.

My co-chair gave me the sign that it was time to end the conversation. I told John we were going to have to continue with the auction. I said "John, before you hang up. . . there's one thing I have to know. Do you have freckles?" He began to laugh.

"Oh, yes. I have freckles all over...all over."

"I knew it," I yelled. I put my hand over the mouthpiece of the phone. The phone was a two-way speaker phone. Everyone could hear what was being said.

"You guys . . . he has freckles. He has freckles!!"

On March 30, 1990, I received a bone marrow transplant. It gave me new blood, new marrow - it gave me LIFE; and yes. . . *it even gave me freckles!*

In completing the book you are now reading, I began to experience a small amount of anxiety. Each section of this book: <u>Miracles in the Midst of Hell, The Child Within</u> and <u>Celebrate Life</u>, is dedicated to a person I have grown to love in a very special way. I never got to meet these people who have so touched my life.

I placed a phone call to Arlene Leibs. She is the mother of David Leibs, who <u>The Child Within</u> is dedicated to. We are good friends. I absolutely adore the woman. We decided to meet for lunch. She was going to bring David's picture with her. I would use it for the book in dedication. I was so excited about seeing her. She cried when she spoke of David. David was not able to find a donor. He was never given a chance to have a transplant. She gave me the letter she had written for David's eulogy. It reads as follows:

*David Leibs our beloved son died February 2, 1990 at Baylor Hospital in Dallas, Texas.*

*He was born and raised in Dallas. He was a sweet, gentle loving boy.*

*He lost his valiant fight with leukemia. He was courageous throughout the long 18 month battle.*

*We were blessed with "grace periods," during that time, given to us through the intervention of medicine and good doctors. Periods of time when David was feeling well and looking well and in good spirits. He made it easier on us who had to stand by and watch.*

*We thank God and are so grateful for His giving us those special times.*

*We thank God for letting us have our David for 33 years.*

*We will miss all of the many more years he should have had to be shared with us, his loving family.*

*David always believed in tomorrow. That there would still be another medicine and that a cure would be found in his lifetime. Please God, a cure will be found soon for all the other leukemia patients.*

*It was his fervent wish to see his "little girls" Marissa 5 and Kera 3 "grow up." He said he would be real tough on the guys who came to date them. He remembered what he was like, as a boy, taking girls out.*

*He loved rain and snow, boating, skiing, camping in Colorado and animals.*

*He fell in love with his wife Elisa at first sight.*

*His sister Janis adored him and his brother Louis thought he was about the best guy in the world. They were very special to each other.*

*Our hearts are broken with his loss but we will keep him alive in our hearts and in our mind forever.*

*We will keep him alive in our wonderful memories of him.*

*He was our baby.*
*He is our Beloved David.*
*He will always be loved.*

*Arlene and Jerry Leibs*
*February 1990*

Arlene wrote that just a few days following David's death. As we talked about David, she said that it was still very difficult for her. "I couldn't say that for a long time. . . that David had *died*." We searched for other things to discuss. It seemed the only thing that continued to surface was cancer, death, transplants, fund raising. . we had nothing else to say.

As we talked, Arlene reached out and touched my hand. "Christine, I hear about you doing all these things because people tell me. I know that you are always running to Metro Medical and visiting with patients. You send cards and letters. And you call those that are going to have a transplant. And you're working with Life-Link and you're doing fund-raising. And you're writing this book. . . and that's all good. You are doing a lot, but Sweet-heart, what I don't hear is what you are doing for Christine." I just looked at her. I could feel the sting from the words that she spoke to me.

"Christine, no matter how much you do and no matter how much you try and accomplish, Sweet-heart, you can't bring David back from the dead. David is dead. You are right. . . I believe that David is still alive and he will always live in our hearts, but Christine, I can't touch him. And I can't feel him, but I can touch you. You have been given *YOUR LIFE* and you need to get on with the business of living it." She then reached out and touched the front cover of the manuscript. She said this book is good and you need to finish it. But, Christine, when it is complete, you need to close the book and go on with your life. You've been given life and you need to enjoy it." She patted the cover of the book. "This can be part of it, but it can't be all of it."

That meeting was two weeks ago. As I went home I knew that Arlene had spoken the truth. I had become extremely uncomfortable in social situations. It seemed as though everywhere I went. . . I never fit in. The thing that I sought all of my life was to be accepted for who I was. But now I was hiding behind a mask again: Christine - the cancer survivor.

"Oh, *you're* Christine Michael. I have heard so much about you. It such an honor to meet you." My cancer would be the topic of discussion no matter where I went. After attending an event that was purely social, I realized how true it was. It was as if I were on center stage. I discovered that unless I was talking about my cancer, I had nothing to say. I had fought so hard to live. Now, living my life had become the thing that I fought against the most. I fought with everything inside of me to get away from cancer. Now my entire identity was labeled "cancer survivor."

I realized much of what I was doing was being motivated by survivor's guilt. And I never knew it. I had an earnest desire to help others. Yet, if I could not help them, I was miserable. My days were filled with guilt. It was impossible for me to be at peace. I had taken it on as my personal responsibility to save all of the cancer patients from dying. I was so fortunate to be alive. But underneath. . . I still have the same child within that struggles daily. It is an everyday battle with me to feel good about myself. . . to feel that I deserve to be happy.

Two weeks after my lunch with Arlene, I received a note from her. It read:

*Dear Christine:*

*The loss of a loved one is devastating. You never really get over it, but you find a way to go on because you have to. You count your blessings and thank God for what you do have.*
*You have been **given** your life from someone who had the heart to care for another human being whom they didn't even know and never met. Use your life as it was intended. Reach out instead of back and find the joy there is. Put "life" back into living.*
*You will always do "good things" and want to be involved in some way with furthering the efforts to help leukemia patients but do that in addition to your life; not instead of it. Get out and get involved with the business of living life to its fullest.*

*Love,*
*Arlene*

I thought about the verse in the Bible I had struggled with for so many years. I always thought I knew what it meant. . . . "These things I have spoken to you, that your joy may be made full. My joy is in you.

Greater love has no one than those who lay down their life for his friends." I had tried for months to "lay down my life" for my friends. . . there are so many that need help. There are so many that are dying.

I thought about the night before I had my transplant. The only thing that I had to hold on to was Christopher Michael saying "Mommy, please don't give up. Please fight for me." I saw so many children's faces that said, "We can't fight. Please fight for us." That is what I had been trying to do.

Arlene was right. I had been trying to bring David back from the dead. I was going to lay down my life so David could still live. I thought if I could keep others from dying - then the ones that didn't make it could still be with us. But somehow, David, who laid down his life and went to be with God, was giving my life back to me. Life really does go on. It's a circle that cannot be broken.

After struggling for a couple of days, I decided that I needed to face my pain. As I picked up the manuscript to begin writing, I burst into tears. I saw the cover that read: "By Christine Michael." I realized that there was more than just my cancer and my guilt about being alive when so many others have died - that I was not letting go of. . .

My name is not Christine Michael. My name is Norma. Christopher Michael was my son. And he died. I wanted that baby more than anything in this world. I wrote Christopher Michael a letter. I tried to start it numerous times, but I couldn't go through with it. I couldn't face the fact that Christopher Michael was not coming back.

Today is September 2, 1991. Christopher Michael would have been three-years-old today had he lived. Or would he? Was my baby born on that day or did he die on that day? I woke up at 2:00 A.M. on September 4, 1991 and began to write:

*9/3/91*

*Dear Christopher Michael:*

*It's 2:00 A.M. I guess it's actually September 4. How ironic. . . I just realized it has been one year exactly since your daddy and I were legally deemed 'null and void'.. One year ago today our marriage was annulled. ..I was so in love with your father, Christopher Michael. I had taken my vows until "death do us part." I couldn't go through with a divorce. Now I look back and think "What difference does it make?" No matter what you call it, it is still the same thing. Your daddy and I aren't together and we will never be again. I've dealt with that and I've released your daddy in my heart. He was a good man, Christopher Michael. He had been real hurt. You don't know what that is. And I'm real thankful for that. I'm thankful that all you will know is happiness and joy. You know, Baby, I still love your daddy. I'll always love him. I've gone on with my life... I thought I was doing great. So much has happened in just one week. I was on the last chapter of my book when I met with Arlene. That's David's mommy. You need to get to know him. I've never met him but I know he is very special. He helped me get back on the path to living last week. He lives in his mommy's heart just like you live in mine.*

*I've spent half of the week running from having to face you, Christopher Michael. I don't want to let you go. The pain is so deep in my heart and it hurts so badly. Yesterday, you would have been three years old: September 2, 1991. That was your great grandmother's birthday. My heart still breaks when I think about that day. Christopher Michael, when the nurse came to take me to Labor and Delivery, I literally thought I was going to die. My heart still aches. I wanted you so badly. A part of me wanted to die that day. I think a part of me did die, Baby. I can still remember what if felt like to have you move inside of me. . . to lie down at night and to feel you kick. That has got to be the most incredible feeling in the world.*

*I had bought you a little blue bib outfit. It had a baseball cap with it. The words "Home-run Baby" was written across the top. That's how I told your daddy that I was pregnant. I laid the outfit on his pillow with a card. I don't know how I knew you were a little boy. I just always knew. I always looked at "little boy" clothes. When I bought the furniture for your room downstairs I decorated it in blue. I still have the wallpaper up. I never changed it. It has little "teddy bears" on it. The border paper says "I love my teddy bear. My teddy bear loves me. Everywhere I go, my teddy bear goes with me."*

*Baby, I don't want to let you go. It's just so hard. It took me until February to even admit that you existed. Christopher Michael, you are the only thing that kept me alive...I couldn't stand losing you. I couldn't stand the thought of having you come through the birth canal dead. Now I would give anything to know what you looked like. I have a description. You were a little longer than one foot in length. I've gotten a ruler out so many times and tried to see you in it. You weighed 24 ounces...You were my perfect little boy. You had 10 fingers and 10 toes. . .perfect. except you died.*

*It's hard to let you go because I don't know if yesterday was your birthday or if it was the day that you died. I still think about January 3. That was the day you were due to be born.*
*I am so angry with your father. I feel like when he left me. . .he took you with him. And that hurts so desperately in knowing that he never really even wanted you. I would never tell you that if you were alive, Baby. He use to get so angry with me when I cried after losing you. He wanted to bury it and pretend you never existed.*

*He left me so I could have the children that I always wanted. I was devastated. I relapsed with leukemia 3 months later. I'm now told that I am sterile for life. I'll never be able to have another child. When Dr. Duckett came to tell me that you had died, he said, "You'll never be able to replace this one, but in a couple of years, after the sterility effects of your chemotherapy wears off, you can try again." I never wanted to try again. I wanted you.*

*I finally reached a point that I did want to have another baby. Your dad and I were going to try again in December. But Duckett was right. Nothing will ever replace Christopher Michael. .*

*Christopher Michael, I thought I could hold on to you through your father. He knew what you looked like and as long as I had him. . . I had you. When he left - he took you with him.*
*I guess that's because in reality. . . I never really had you. You didn't live, Christopher Michael. You weren't born. You died. You had a life but it was inside of me. And that's where you have been ever since. . . inside of me.*

*I have spent my life in the last three years trying to bring you back. I have cried and agonized over all of the children that are dying from cancer because. . . in every one of them - I see you. Or the face that I created in my mind for you.*

*You're not coming back. . . are you, Christopher Michael? You weren't really ever here to come back. No matter how many people I talk with, how many speaking engagements I do or how many funds I raise. . . you're not coming back. And I have to accept that.*

*I have got to quit living my life through you. I can't keep you alive by helping to get more people in the bone marrow registry. You are dead, Sweet-heart. It has taken me 3 years to say that. You will always live in my heart.*

*People don't understand what it is like to lose a child - especially when you are told that you can never have another. Baby, I have to release you. I have got to let you go. You have been my entire life - my only reason for existing. But I have got to go on with my life. I can't touch you. I can't hold you. No matter how much I hold on to your memory - it's not going to change the fact that you are gone. All I have left is the pain and I've got to let it go.*

*Christopher Michael, I love you with all my heart. I believe that you are alive and that someday I will hold you.*

*There is so much that I need to know. I cry when I think about you facing death. You were alone. I always wondered if you were afraid. Did you know what was happening? I have beaten myself up for choosing to not see you. I just wish I could have held you. But you weren't even there - were you? You were already gone.*

*It's so hard for me to say this because I feel like I'm leaving you. I feel like I am abandoning you. But Christopher Michael, I have got to go with my own life. God has given me life and I haven't lived it since I lost you. I threw myself into your daddy when you died. When he left. . . I threw myself into working with cancer patients.*

*As Arlene so delicately told me at lunch last week, "You can't bring David back" and I can't bring you back. I thought that if I could help save others from dying than I could keep you alive. It just doesn't work that way, Baby. I can't touch you and I can't feel you, but there are some children that I* **can** *touch and that I can feel. As you showed me in such a special way. . . they* **do** *need help. They can't fight for themselves.*

*I can't save them, but I can help them. I, along with the help of many others, can fight for them. They aren't you. But they are alive and they deserve a chance to live.*

*I love you, Christopher Michael. Your mommy is going on with her life. I will always love you. You will always live within my heart. I need for you to understand that it is time; if there was anything that I could do to bring you back. . . I would do it. But there is not.*

*I am releasing you, Christopher Michael. You can run and play and live your new life with all the other children in Heaven. Be sure and get to know David Mayo, David Leibs and Ashley Bradford.*

*Your mommy is going to learn how to play too. I went to swing on the swing-set at the park this week. There's a little child inside of me that needs to learn how to live again.*

*Baby, I don't know exactly how it works up there. But if you can. . . would you ask God to help heal the pain of the people left down here? So many people have a secret place in their heart that no one sees.*

*It's time for all of us to learn to Celebrate Life! I'm going to do that, Sweet-heart. My life begins today. You are my precious son.*

*I will always love you.
One day I will hold you but until then. . . you will always be in my heart.
I'm going to learn how to live again. I'm going to learn how to laugh again. Not just on the outside but on the inside too.*

*It's time to Celebrate Life, Baby.
I love you.
Goodbye Christopher Michael
I love you
Mommy*                         *Dated: 9/4/91  4:06 A.M.*

I could tell after writing the letter I still had not released the pain. I had named my pain. I have faced my pain and embraced it. But I had not let it go. I heard the voice within me say, "Norma, life goes on. Celebrate Life."

The Balloons! I thought about the balloons and about the balloon ride journey we took at the party. That was it! I had some balloons left over from the "Celebrate Life" Party. That was my answer. But where would I go?

Being on a "take care of Norma" kick, I rolled out of bed, threw on a pair of "sweats" and went to walk in the park. I walked three miles when I found my answer. I had completely blocked the place out of my memory. The night I was diagnosed with leukemia, Dr. Duckett told Joe and I about a place on the roof of Dallas Community Hospital. We had gone up there to be alone. We cried together and talked to Christopher Michael.

During my walk, I heard a voice say "Go to the source of your pain." That roof-top is where I left my pain. When I lost my baby. . . a part of me died that night. I began to have flashbacks about the day in Labor and Delivery. Besides Joe, Dr. Duckett and Diane -Dr. Duckett's nurse - were the only people that knew what Christopher Michael looked like. I knew I had to go there and face my pain.

I called Diane and told her what was happening. She was at the "Celebrate Life" party, so she knew the significance of the balloons. I made arrangements to meet her in Labor and Delivery at 11:00 P.M. That is when she got off work. She was going to walk me through my pain. I arrived at the hospital at 10:00 P.M. I knew that I would have to get there early to get my nerve up to go inside. As I was sitting in my car, I saw "Ducky" (Dr.Duckett) getting into his car. I jumped out of my car to meet him. Within seconds he said, "Well, hi" and came over to give me a hug.

"Did you bring your balloons?" he asked.

"Yeah. They're in the car," I said. I was some-what embarrassed and felt a little foolish bringing 12 helium balloons to Labor and Delivery. I had each one blown up. There was one of every color. Each balloon had a different color ribbon tied to it. I could only find one that had the words "Celebrate Life" printed on it. I later realized that was Christopher Michael's balloon. The rest were for me.

I bought a baby-blue candy cane that said "It's a Boy" on it. It was tied to the balloon. I also had a bright yellow card attached. It said: "Tonight I celebrate my life by releasing the following things to God. . . Christopher Michael. Open your arms, Baby, here they come! I accept your death by releasing these balloons." The other side of the card said "Tonight I Celebrate my life by receiving the following things from God. . . *MY LIFE!* My happiness. My health and well-being. By releasing these balloons - I choose to go on."

After Duckett left, I called Labor and Delivery from my car phone. I knew that Diane would wonder if I was still coming. We had not talked since Thursday. We had just planned to meet at 11:00 P.M. More than that, though, I called so I would not "chicken out." At 10:59 P.M. my heart began to beat rapidly. I had broken out in a rash earlier that evening due to nervousness. I told myself, "Norma, just get out of the car and go do it. Face your pain. Get it out. Your freedom is just on the other side." At 11:00 P.M. I got out of my car, locked the door and headed toward the entrance of the hospital. I could feel my legs shaking beneath me as I approached the door - the door that led to the place where I lost something that was irreplaceable. I knew that when I entered that door, I was going to have to face the pain that almost killed me. Even worse, I knew I had nothing to hold on to this time. There would be no future baby. I was sterile. The hormones that I had taken after my transplant caused my cycle to stop completely. All I had was myself.

As I got closer to the entrance, I remembered how close that Labor and Delivery was to the parking lot. Once I entered the door. . . there was no turning back. I heard a voice within me say: "Gut it out, Norma. Face it. You won't have to do this again. You're almost there."

I felt a bit silly carrying in 12 helium balloons to Labor and Delivery. As I sat in the car waiting for the clock to change to 11:00 P.M., I thought about what I was going to say if someone asked me about the balloons. I could see someone saying "Oh, look at all of the balloons. Did someone just have a baby?"

I would say: "Yeah. I did - three years ago. He died." Thinking about that scenario made me want to start the car and go home. I am so thankful I did not leave. As I entered the building I saw the waiting room that I had just pictured in my mind minutes before. No one was there except for the faces in my memory.

The hall was quiet. The building appeared to be totally empty. I mustered up the courage to open the door with the words that hurt so deeply: *Labor and Delivery*. I entered to find Diane coming around the corner.

"Hi, Sweetie," she said. "Are you all ready for this?" she asked as she gave me a hug.

"No," I said. "I'm not. I really don't want to do this."

"Well, you don't have to," she said. "Are you sure?"

"No," I said. "I definitely want to do it. I've got to do it. I've got to go on with my life. I'm just not looking forward to it."

Diane was exactly who I needed that night. She had been by my side the entire time during labor and delivery. It was her day off, but she had come to be with me. Duckett had done the same. They both stayed in Delivery with me until Dr. Duckett took me to CCU. Now Diane was by my side once again.

It was so special to share that night with her, and spend a few poignant moments with "Ducky." The only people that knew what Christopher Michael looked like - apart from Joe - shared the most special moment of my life with me . . . telling him good-bye.

"Is anyone here?" I asked. "It's so quiet."

"No. Just you. I took the last mother up to her room right before you got here. It's all yours," she said. We walked past the nurse's station to the first labor room. Diane grabbed my hand. "This is where you were," she said.

I put my hand over my mouth. Tears pooled in my eyes. I could see myself lying on the table - paralyzed. I could see the IV poles with the chemotherapy, antibiotics and other medications attached. I could smell the smell of death in the room from that night. It was difficult for me to not turn my head in horror.

"Do you remember what Joe was doing?" I asked.

"I don't remember anything about Joe. All I remember is that he was just so quiet. He wouldn't talk to anybody. It's like he wasn't even there that night. I can't even picture his face being in the room that night," Diane said.

I smiled as I thought, "That's because he really *wasn't* there. He was already gone, too. There was no life inside of Joe." I took one last look at the room. I closed my eyes and allowed myself to feel the pain.

"I wanted to die that night, Diane" I said. "I think a part of me did die. I wanted Christopher Michael more than anything in this world." Tears ran down my face. "It's just so hard to let go."

I looked up into her eyes that were filled with tears.

"Do you want to go to delivery?" Diane asked.

"Yes, I do. I need to," I said.

We went to the dressing room so I could change clothes. I put on my scrubs. As we approached the delivery room, Diane said, "This is where you were." I had trouble looking into the room.

"You probably don't remember this," she said.

"Yeah I do. I remember coming down the hall." My heart was aching as I talked about it. "I remember Joe was wearing his blue scrubs. He was holding my hand. He looked so handsome." Joe had majored in Pre-Med and had planned on going to medical school. He was going to be a medical missionary. "I remember looking at him and thinking 'You would have made such a wonderful doctor.' Then I remember thinking, 'Oh God, I want to die - but I am so in love with Joe.' I couldn't stand to be awake. And that's all I remember."

Diane and I never went into the delivery room. The door was wide open. We just stood outside and looked in. I think that is because I realized there was nothing there to see. Christopher Michael had come into this world in that room - my son was dead. As I looked into the same room that had held the most precious thing in my life. . . it was cold and sterile. There was no life in it. I felt detached from that room. Nothing seemed familiar. I thought that I would find Christopher Michael there - but suddenly I realized - he was truly gone.

I had faced my biggest fear. It was the deepest pain of my life. But when I dared to look within and to face the pain that almost killed me, I realized that the pain was the only thing left. It was over. All I had to do was to let go of it.

Diane was talking to me as we walked toward the recovery room. I was deep in thought and still trying to process everything that was happening. As we went in the room Diane said, "Now I don't remember where you were in here."

"I do," I said immediately. "I was right there." I pointed to the right-hand side of the room. It was the second table. "No one else was in here. I remember you and 'Ducky' were at the desk across from me." "I remember "Ducky" taking me to CCU," I continued. "He didn't leave my side until I fell asleep." I thought about the nurse in CCU that asked me where my baby was. And I thought about waking up in the middle of the night with milk seeping from my breasts - ready to feed Christopher Michael.

"Diane, what did he look like?" I asked as I was staring off remembering that moment. I looked over at her. "Do you remember? Joe said there was something wrong with his mouth. That it wasn't completely formed?"

"There was nothing wrong with his mouth!" Diane said. "He was very blue, which is normal since he had died. He was completely formed and fully developed. He was *little* because he was so young."

"The autopsy said that he was a little more than a foot long," I said as I tried to help her see him more clearly. She didn't need any help though. Diane was my friend. She was the first one that had gotten to me when I checked into my room. She was there before Joe. She was the one that sat on my bed and cried be-cause my baby had died. She remembered Christopher Michael clearly.

She measured with her hands what she estimated to be a foot long. "Yeah. That's about right. Maybe a little longer; probably about 15 inches. But he had hands with little tiny fingers. He had 10 toes. He was a perfect little baby boy."

"What color were his eyes? Or were they closed?" I asked.

"They were closed. I couldn't tell what color they were," she said.

"Most babies are born with blue eyes. Aren't they?"

"Yeah. A kind of slate gray-blue," she said.

We continued to talk as we returned to the delivery room. We went to the lounge where we had left the balloons. As I looked at the one balloon that said "Celebrate Life," I smiled. Just hours before, my heart broke when I looked at that balloon. Now my heart was being filled with warmth. Diane and I started climbing the stairs to the rooftop. We opened the door and it was everything that I had remembered. It was beautiful. You could see for miles. The night was cool and there was a gentle breeze blowing. We walked over to the brick wall that bordered the roof. The wall came a few inches above my waist. As I looked out over the wall, I could see the courtyard of the hospital. Everything was so peaceful and quiet. It was as if there were no one else moving in the world except God, Diane, Christopher Michael and me. The balloons were being beaten by the wind.

"Did he have any hair?" I asked.

"He had peach fuzz," she said.

"What color was it?" I asked. Before she had a chance to answer I said "You know I *never* could talk to Joe about this. He would get so angry with me when I wanted to talk about it."

"It looked like it was dark brown, but it was wet so it could have been lighter. It probably was lighter. Probably about your color," she said.

We stayed on the roof of the hospital until 4:00 A.M. It was where I experienced the deepest pain of my life. I had left Christopher Michael there on September 2, 1988. I didn't carry home a new-born baby boy wrapped up in a blanket like I thought I would. I carried home an empty blanket that was full of pain and death and sadness. Diane and I talked about life and we talked about death. We talked about dreams and heartaches and desires and we shared a special moment. We laughed and we cried. We talked about family and where life begins.

"That's all I ever wanted, Diane. . . to be a mother. Nothing else mattered," I said as I looked onto the hospital grounds. I had been holding those 12 helium balloons for hours. I looked at the one that said "Celebrate Life" and the blue candy-cane that said "It's a Boy."

I wondered if Christopher Michael could see me; if he knew how very much I loved him. I looked at the balloons being tossed in the wind. I looked at my hand that was having to hold them so tightly so they wouldn't blow away. I knew it was time. There was nothing left to hold on to. Everything I needed was right within my own heart. It had been there all along.

I looked up into the sky. The stars were bright and beautiful. I breathed deeply, wiped the tears from my face and read the card that I had written: "Tonight I celebrate my life by releasing the following things to God. . . Christopher Michael. Open your arms, Baby.

Here they come. I accept your death by releasing these balloons." I turned the card over and read it out loud. "Tonight I celebrate my life by receiving the following things from God. . . .*MY LIFE*!! My happiness, my health, my well-being. I sighed as I finished. . . "By releasing these balloons I choose to go on with my life."

I blew a kiss into the air. "I love you, Christopher Michael. Open your arms, Baby. . here they come." I let go of the balloons. They slowly took off and then started to come back down to the ground.

"Oh no!" I yelled. "They don't want to go. It was hard enough to let go of them the first time. These are for you, Baby!" I hesitated for a moment. ". . . .And it's for me." As I verbalized, "And it's for me. . .", a gust of wind lifted the balloons high above the rooftop. They were being carried into the heavens by the gentle breeze of God.

We watched the balloons fly over the hospital, over the shopping center and far into the night sky. The wind continued to carry them until we could no longer see them. I looked at Diane and smiled. "Three years. . . and all I was holding on to was the pain. I feel so close to him now. All I have is warmth and love." I closed my eyes and put my hand to my chest. I took a deep breath.

". . . AND I HAVE MY LIFE!" I said.

The dawn was quickly approaching. Diane and I had been there most of the night. As I think about Christopher Michael now, all I see is happiness. Where there was pain - there is now peace. Before, the only thing I had were the memories that I created in my mind. Now. . ..I have the beautiful sight of Christopher Michael being lifted by the gentle breeze into the hands of God.

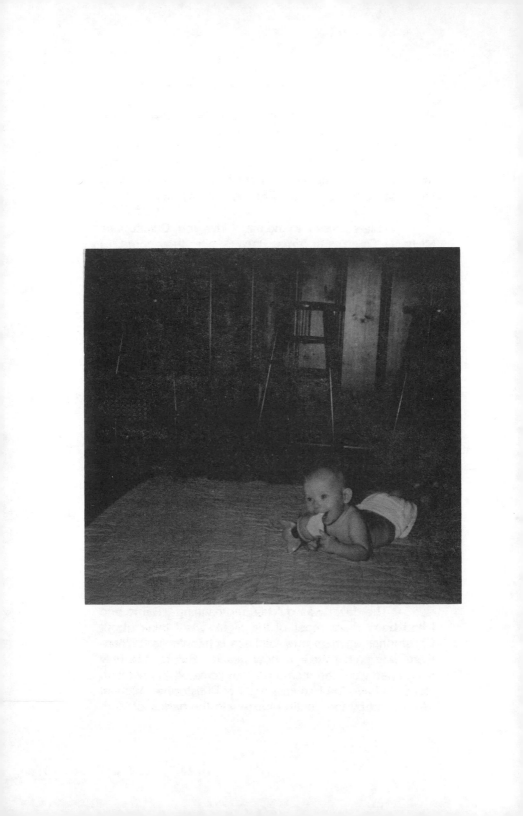

I hope you get well.
I hope your trip is safe when you go home.
I love you.
Love,
Trae

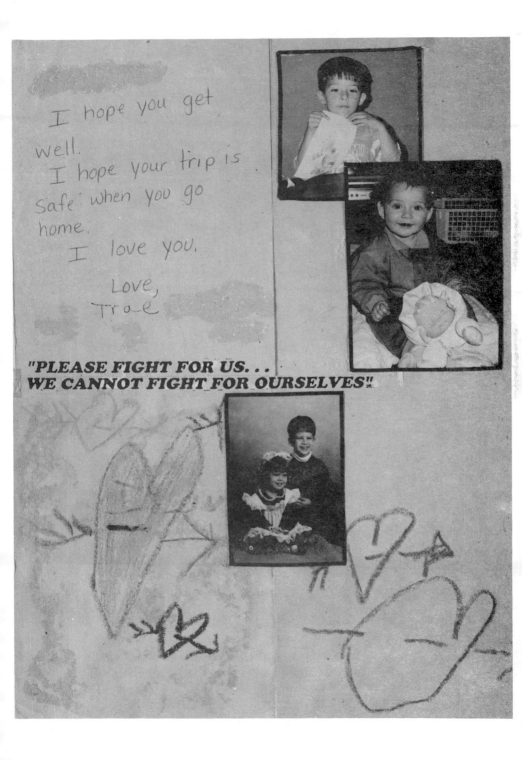

**"PLEASE FIGHT FOR US. . .**
**WE CANNOT FIGHT FOR OURSELVES"**

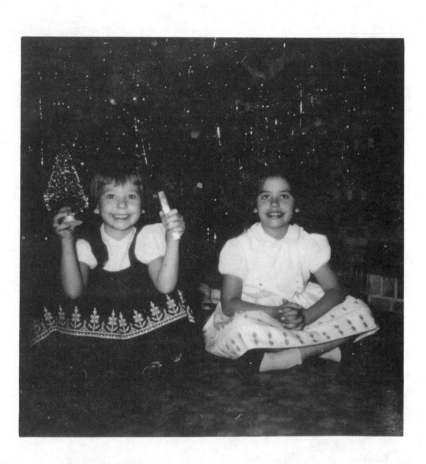

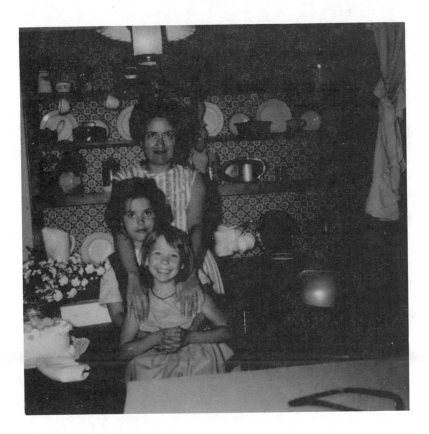

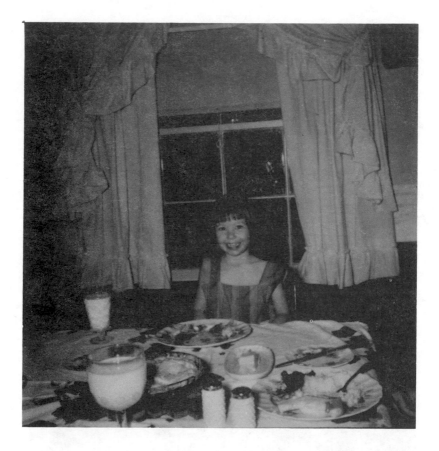

# CHAPTER EIGHT

## On to the Mountain Top

The following week, I left for what the National Geographic calls "one of the ten most beautiful views of the world.". . . the Mountain Top in St. Thomas, Virgin Islands. Three years ago I thought I lived on the mountain top. Now the view is so much more beautiful. I now see further and I see deeper than I have ever seen before. I look at my life before this experience. My view of life and my perception of "hell" was so different. I have since found that ability to feel pain is a precious gift we are given; for without the knowledge of pain we would never understand the reality of a blessing. It is through pain that we can reach out and find the ability to overcome.

As I look down at each obstacle I have encountered, I see each experience as a stepping stone to get me to where I am today. I have lost everything a person can lose in this lifetime, but what I have been given is so much more precious than any thing I ever had. I am no longer searching. I am no longer climbing to reach the top. That void is now filled. It is filled with something, that to my surprise, was there all the time. It is filled with a God who loves me and who has given me the dignity and the freedom to search within my own heart for the faith and the peace to celebrate life as I view it. It has been that way from the beginning. He made me a precious child. He gave me the parents He wanted me to have and He made me exactly as He wanted me to be. The answer was there all the time.

I have been to the valley and I have been to the mountain top. But the beautiful view comes from having the courage to look within. It is there our path is defined. Even in the valley of despair, it is within our own hearts we find the mountain top. Only then. . . can we begin to celebrate life each and every day.

*You do not need to be loved*
*Not at the cost of losing yourself*
*The single relationship that is truly central and assured*
*in life is the relation to the self.*
*It is rewarding to find someone that you like,*
*but it is indispensable to view yourself*
*as acceptable.*
*It is a delight to discover people who are worthy*
*of respect, admiration and love*
*but it is vital to believe in yourself as deserving of these*
*things*
*For you cannot live in someone else*
*You cannot find yourself in someone else*
*For all the people that you will know in a lifetime*
*You are the only one you will never leave or lose*
*To the questions in your life*
*You are the answer*
*To the problems in your life*
*You are the solution*
*[Anonymous]*

My prayer is that every person who goes through the struggle of cancer. . . or the heartbreak of an ended marriage. . . or the devastation of losing a child, will search within themselves to find the answers. As human beings we have a tendency to search outside of ourselves to find the reasons for life's events. What I have found is the answer lies within ourselves. It's within our own heart that we find peace. It only comes from within.

It was a beautiful experience when I realized the thing I had searched for all my life was right within my own heart. It was in learning to love myself that I found the happiness I had been missing throughout my existence. I thought Joe and Christopher Michael could fulfill that empty place deep within my heart. I discovered that the mountain top I was always strived to reach. . .

I had already arrived.  I had been there all along and I never even knew it.  It was in taking off the masks that I began to see the beautiful life God had given me.  It was when I began to believe in myself. . . . I knew everything I needed would be provided for me.  I didn't have to seek.  I only had to believe.

I no longer have to look down or look back with regrets.  I can begin to live each and every day on the mountain top.  I can celebrate the life that God gave me when he breathed life into my existence.  It was what He was trying to tell me many months ago. . . "you are the master of your own destiny.  You determine the delineation of your faith.  It has been that way from the beginning."

Whatever it is that is in your heart. . . in that little secret place that no one sees - right now is the best time to let it go.  Whether it is the death of a child, the devastation of a broken relationship, the love you never received from a parent. . . whatever it is that is weighing your life down. . . it is time for each of us to let it go. As we finish this chapter together. . . you in reading it and I in writing it, it is time to close the book and put it on the shelf.  Today is the day that we can begin to celebrate the life that God has given us.  He has made you special and unique.  There is not another person on this entire Earth like yourself.  You are the best <u>YOU</u> you can be!  Believe it!  I invite you to join me in completing this book.  No one has to know.  Close your eyes and allow yourself to feel the love that you deserve.  Have the courage to look within and see the precious child that God made you.

Allow yourself to receive whatever it is that you are in need of. . . love, peace, acceptance, forgiveness for yourself, a healing, whatever it is. . . the deepest desires of your heart are there to be met.  Attach them to your balloon and let them go.

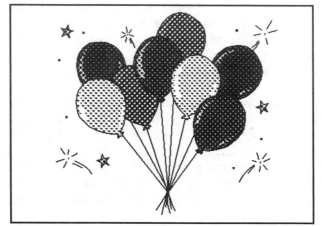

## *Tonight I Celebrate My Life by Releasing the following things to God. . .*

## *Tonight I Celebrate My Life by Receiving the following things from God. . .*

And begin to celebrate life. You are precious. You are special and you are loved *just as you are.* It's time to take the masks off. The answer is within your own heart. As you find it and finish this chapter. . .close the book, put it on the shelf and "get on with the business of living."

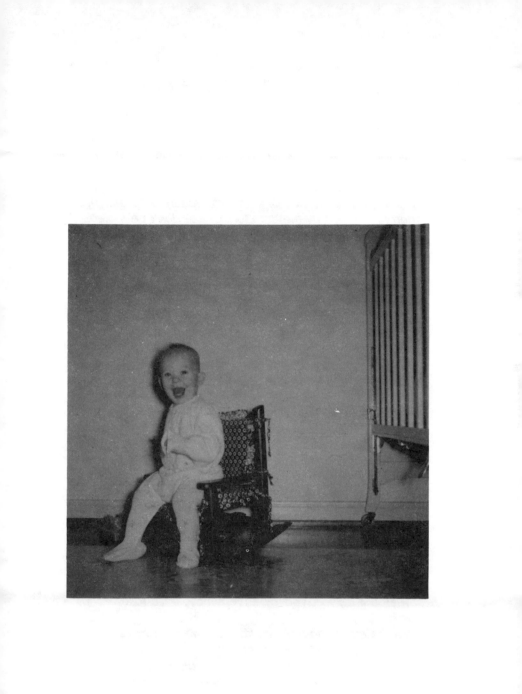

# PLEASE HEAR WHAT I'M NOT SAYING

*Don't be fooled by me*
*Don't be fooled by the face I wear*
*For I wear a mask, I wear a thousand masks, masks that*
*I am afraid to take off*
*and none of them are me.*
*Pretending is an art that's second nature with me, but*
*don't be fooled by me, for God's sake don't be fooled.*
*I give you the impression that I'm secure,*
*that all is sunny and unruffled with me,*
*Within as well as without*
*that confidence is my name and coolness my game, that*
*the waters calm and I'm in command, and I need no one.*
*But don't believe me.*
*Please!*
*My surface may seem smooth, but my surface is my*
*mask,*
*My ever-varying and ever-concealing mask.*
*Beneath lies no smugness; no complacence*
*Beneath dwells the real me in confusion, in fear, in*
*aloneness*
*But I hide this*
*I don't want anybody to know it.*
*I panic at the thought of my weakness and fear being*
*exposed.*
*That's why I frantically create a mask to hide behind,*
*A nonchalant, sophisticated facade, to help me pretend*
*to shield me from the glance that knows.*
*But such a glance is precisely my salvation, my only*
*salvation.*
*And I know it.*
*That is if it's followed by acceptance, if it's followed by*
*love.*
*It's the only thing that can liberate me from myself;*
*from my own self-built prison walls,*
*from the barriers that I so painstakingly erect.*
*It's the only thing that will assure me of what I can't*
*assure myself. . . that I really am worth something.*

*But I don't tell you this. I don't dare.*

I'm afraid to, I'm afraid you'll think less of me, that you'll laugh, and your laugh would kill me.
I'm afraid that deep down I'm nothing, that I'm just no good.
And that you will see this and reject me.
So I play my game, my desperate pretending game with a facade of assurance without, and a trembling child within.
And so begins the parade of masks, the glittering but empty parade of masks
and my life becomes a front
I idly chatter to you in suave tones of surface talk.
I tell you everything that's really nothing
and nothing of what's everything, of what's crying within me.

So when I'm going through my routine do not be fooled by what I'm saying
Please listen carefully and try to hear what I'm not saying
What I'd like to be able to say, what for survival I need to say,
But I can't say.
I dislike hiding. Honestly.
I dislike the superficial game I'm playing, superficial phony game.
I'd really like to be genuine and spontaneous, and me,
But you've got to help me
I've got to hold your hand,
Even when that's the last thing I seem to want or need.
Only you can wipe away from my eyes the blank stare of breathing dead.
Only you can call me into aliveness.
Each time you're kind, and gentle, and encouraging,
Each time you try to understand
because you really care
My heart begins to grow wings, very small wings
very feeble wings, but wings.
With your sensitivity and sympathy, and your power of understanding
You breathe life into me. I want you to know how important you are to me
how you can be a

*Creator of the person that is me if you choose to*
*Please choose to.*

*You alone can break down the wall behind which I*
*tremble.*
*You alone can remove my mask*
*You alone can release me from my shadow world of*
*panic, uncertainty*
*From my lonely prison.*
*Do not pass me by. Please do not pass me by.*
*It will not be easy for you.*
*A long conviction of worthlessness build strong walls.*
*The nearer you approach to me, the blinder I may strike*
*back.*
*It's irrational, but despite what the books say*
*about me, I am irrational. I fight against the very thing I*
*want.*
*But I am told that*
*Love is stronger than walls, and in this lies my hope.*
*My only hope.*

*Please try to beat down those walls with firm hands*
*But with gentle hands.*
*For a child is very sensitive.*
*Who am I, you may wonder?*
*I am someone you know very well.*
*For I am every man you meet and I am every woman you*
*meet.*                    *-Anonymous-*